THE CARING SELF

A volume in the series
The Culture and Politics of Health Care Work
edited by Suzanne Gordon and Sioban Nelson

A list of titles in this series is available at
www.cornellpress.cornell.edu.

The Caring Self

The Work Experiences of Home Care Aides

Clare L. Stacey

ILR Press
an imprint of
Cornell University Press
Ithaca and London

First published 2011 by Cornell University Press
First printing, Cornell Paperbacks, 2011

Printed in the United States of America

Library of Congress Cataloging-in-Publication Data

Stacey, Clare L. (Clare Louise), 1973–
    The caring self : the work experiences of home care aides /
Clare L. Stacey.
        p. cm. — (The culture and politics of health care work)
    Includes bibliographical references and index.
    ISBN 978-0-8014-4985-7 (cloth : alk. paper) —
    ISBN 978-0-8014-7699-0 (pbk. : alk. paper)
    1. Home health aides—United States.   2. Home care services—
Social aspects—United States.   3. Home care services—United
States—Psychological aspects.   I. Title.   II. Series: Culture and politics
of health care work.
    RA645.35.S68   2011
    362.14—dc22   2010052641

Cornell University Press strives to use environmentally responsible suppliers and materials to the fullest extent possible in the publishing of its books. Such materials include vegetable-based, low-VOC inks and acid-free papers that are recycled, totally chlorine-free, or partly composed of nonwood fibers. For further information, visit our website at www.cornellpress.cornell.edu.

Cloth printing   10 9 8 7 6 5 4 3 2 1
Paperback printing   10 9 8 7 6 5 4 3 2 1

For my parents

Contents

Acknowledgments

Meeting and talking to nursing aides over the last ten years has given me a very real appreciation of what it means to care for another person. Watching aides interact with elderly or disabled clients opened my eyes to the stresses associated with care, and also convinced me that caregiving—especially when carried out in the right conditions—can affirm social ties and give lives meaning, whether we are on the giving or receiving end. I am indebted to the paid caregivers who agreed to talk with me and share their daily experiences. I thank them for opening up their homes and sites of work, and for their candor in talking about both the rewards and constraints of the job. It is my hope that the reading public will take note of their stories and begin to question the low wages and lack of labor protections afforded these workers.

In writing this book, I benefited from the care and support of many people. At the University of California-Davis, mentors, friends, and colleagues read through rough drafts, listened to inchoate ideas, and supported me unconditionally, even during my most neurotic and disorganized moments.

Many faculty members were instrumental in guiding me through graduate school, including Carole Joffe, Debora Paterniti, John Hall, and Mary R. Jackman. I am particularly grateful to Vicki Smith and Ming-Cheng Lo for their advice and encouragement. Thanks also to Janet Gouldner and the editorial collective of *Theory and Society* for keeping me on my toes. My writing group pals, Jeff Sweat and Anna Muraco, saw me through the dissertation year, while Andreana Clay, Magdi Vanya, and Zach Schiller sustained me with friendship and critical conversation. For helping me gain access to home care workers, I thank the many supervisors and administrators at In-Home Supportive Services (IHSS), as well as the social workers and public health nurses who allowed me to shadow and interview them. I also wish to acknowledge the Institute for Research on Labor and Employment at UC Berkeley for granting me a dissertation-year fellowship in 2003–4.

My postdoctoral years at the Institute for Health Policy Studies at UC San Francisco provided me with a strong foundation in health policy, training that helped me think through the wider implications of my findings. Marty Otanez and Stuart Henderson helped me adjust to post-doc life and modeled how to balance the career of a scholar with the joys and challenges of being a parent. While at UCSF I also had the good fortune to work with Daniel Dohan, a mentor who convinced me that medical sociologists can and must make their work relevant beyond academia. Dan also gave me considerable time to be with my child, Lily, after she was born, no questions asked. For that, I am forever grateful.

To my colleagues at Kent State University, thank you for giving me the encouragement and resources to complete this book. Richard Serpe championed the project from day one, while Kristen Marcussen, Dave Purcell, Susan Roxburgh, Manacy Pai, Kelly MacArthur, and André Christi-Mizell offered good humor and unwavering support. Special thanks go to Joanna Dreby, who provided constructive feedback on early drafts, and Jerry Lewis, who reassured me that I was doing things right. Several graduate students lent hours of their labor to transcribing interviews and editing the manuscript. For their dedication and attention to detail, I thank Lindsey Ayers, Christi Gross, and Timothy Adkins. I also appreciate the gift of time (in the form of a research leave) given to me by the Division of Research and Graduate Studies at Kent State during the fall of 2008.

I consider myself lucky to have support networks that seem to hold up well against time and distance. Sarah Fenstermaker inspired me to become a sociologist during my undergraduate years at UC Santa Barbara, and she remains an invaluable mentor. I am also humbled by the exceptional scholars I have met via the Carework Network, who continually push me to think more critically about my arguments. There are too many names to mention here, but I would be remiss if I didn't at least acknowledge Mignon Duffy, Amy Armenia, Mary Tuominen, Ellen Scott, Teresa Scherzer, Julie Whitaker, Mary K. Zimmerman, and Rachel Sherman. At Cornell University Press, the editors and reviewers helped mold my thoughts into a more compelling sociological story. Thanks to Fran Benson, Sioban Nelson, Suzanne Gordon, Katherine Liu, and Eileen Boris for taking my work seriously and for guiding me through the publication process. I also benefited from the professional editorial skills of Veronica Jurgena, whose trained eye improved the manuscript considerably.

Since the early stages of this project, my friends have provided many laughs and much-needed reminders that I shouldn't take myself so seriously. My dear pals in Sacramento sustained me with food, drink, and merriment during the first few years. I am especially thankful to Kim Dochterman and Sarah Singleton, whose stories from the field piqued my sociological interest in home care. In Kent, I benefited from regular and relaxing get-togethers with the children and adults of the Prospect Street community. I feel truly blessed to live among such a wonderful group of people. The children deserve special thanks, for reminding me that a little bit of play every day is absolutely necessary.

I would not have found the courage to finish this project without the love of my family. My parents, Rod and Chris, are to be credited for instilling in me a sense of wonder and for supporting me unconditionally as I discovered my passions. Matt and Helen, my siblings, have politely listened to my sociological rants and have forgiven the time spent away from family gatherings and events. To my family in England, I have fond memories of respites abroad; I hope to return more frequently in the coming years. Closer to home, my daughter, Lily, and my husband, Zach, bore the brunt of the stress that writing a book produces. Lily, mature beyond her years, seemed to know when I needed an extra cuddle or a quiet moment to myself. I thank her for bringing perspective to my life. Zach never wavered in his promise to help me see this through. His patience, brilliant cooking skills, and commitment to a life of balance fueled my productivity and kept me going during the slumps. I treasure our partnership.

Some interview material in the book originally appeared in C. L. Stacey, 2005, "Finding Dignity in Dirty Work: The Constraints and Rewards of Low-Wage Home Care Labour," *Sociology of Health and Illness* 27 (6): 831–54.

THE CARING SELF

INTRODUCTION

On the Front Lines of Care

MR. JONES AND KEISHA

On a warm spring day in April, I accompanied Christina, a white public health nurse, to the home of an elderly African American man who suffers from heart disease, renal failure, diabetes, and mild dementia. Mr. Jones is a seventy-six-year-old man who lives alone in a subsidized housing complex in a low-income suburb of Central City.[1] His only regular visitor is his caregiver Keisha, a young African American woman who is paid to cook, clean, and care for him daily. As we approach his apartment building, Christina is sanguine about Mr. Jones's isolation, recalling that she'd seen much worse while on her religious missions to Zimbabwe and Mozambique years ago.

As we approach Mr. Jones's apartment, Christina motions to be quiet. After standing at Mr. Jones's door for a few minutes, Christina realizes that there is a faint sound coming from the front window of the house. We move toward the sound as Christina calls out Mr. Jones's name loudly. From inside, a man's voice pleads for help. Christina straddles a bush and pushes her face against the closed window. She asks Mr. Jones to unlock the door if he can. Mr. Jones, fatigue in his voice, tells us that he has fallen out of bed and cannot get up. At this moment, we notice a young African American woman coming toward us. She introduces herself as Jodi, the acting "super" of the building. Christina asks Jodi whether she knows Mr. Jones, and she replies, laughing, that of course she knows Mr. Jones. Christina determines that Jodi does not have a key to the apartment but that Keisha, Mr. Jones's home care aide, does. Unfortunately, Jodi has no idea how to reach Keisha.

Christina turns away from the small crowd that has now gathered outside Mr. Jones's apartment, pulls out her cell phone, and dials 911. After about ten minutes, a fire truck pulls up in front of Mr. Jones's apartment. In what seems like seconds, the paramedics are inside the apartment; Christina and I follow close behind. The paramedics, two young men, ask us to wait in the living room while they assess Mr. Jones's condition. From the living room we can hear the paramedics speaking loudly to Mr. Jones, followed by the sound of a collective grunt as the patient is lifted into his wheelchair. Within minutes, Mr. Jones is wheeled out into the living room, where we wait seated on a couch covered with disheveled bed linens.

Seemingly unaware of the commotion surrounding him, Mr. Jones beams at Christina when he sees her. I assume at first that Christina has a well-established rapport with the man, but soon realize his smile is a vacant one, not one of recognition. Christina approaches Mr. Jones and asks him to tell her what happened. Mr. Jones does not respond but stretches out his hand toward Christina. Christina pauses, puts on her rubber gloves, and then takes Mr. Jones by the hand. She again asks what happened, but I can tell from Mr. Jones's singular interest in Christina's face that the trauma of his fall is now a distant memory. The paramedics ask Christina to sign a few papers and then head for the door. As they are leaving, they tell Christina with some condescension to try not to leave Mr. Jones alone in the future. Christina responds by thanking the two paramedics, taking little offense at the misdirected nature of their admonishment.

Once the paramedics clear out, Christina notices that Jodi, the building super, has been standing in the doorway watching events unfold. Jodi nods in the direction of Mr. Jones and says, "Man, those feet are purple." Christina does not respond to Jodi but bends down to examine Mr. Jones's feet, massaging them gently. Mr. Jones laughs aloud, responding to Christina's touch. Christina explains that Mr. Jones is severely dehydrated and is having trouble with his circulation. Jodi adds, unsolicited, that he often falls off his chair at night, which makes things worse.

At that moment Keisha, Mr. Jones's caregiver, walks through the door with a full grocery bag. She appears to be about twenty-five years old. With a passing hello, Keisha walks through the living room into the adjacent kitchen and begins putting away the groceries. With some urgency, Christina tells Keisha what has happened, unsure whether Jodi has been in contact with her. Keisha seems unmoved by Christina's story and confirms Jodi's report that Mr. Jones often falls down when he is alone. Over the clamor of cupboards opening and closing, Keisha elaborates that Mr. Jones insists on trying to reach things—water, books, food—that are not easily within his grasp. When she leaves at night, Keisha puts Mr. Jones into bed and reminds him to stay there. Inevitably, he falls out of bed and cannot get up. I notice that Keisha has a bad head cold and that she looks extremely fatigued. She offers us some instant soup which we decline. What Mr. Jones needs, Keisha explains, is a "grabber," a tool that he can use to reach things at night without endangering himself. She adds that if we really want to solve the problem, we need to get more hours of paid care for Mr. Jones, so that she can watch him at night. Keisha explains that she already works beyond her paid hours for Mr. Jones, staying sometimes until two in the morning without monetary compensation. Keisha explains that Mr. Jones is not very compliant with the social workers and doctors, so they in turn do not help him out much. He badly needs a Lifeline (an emergency call device), Keisha says, but the doctor never filed the approval paperwork to have the device covered by Medicare.

Mr. Jones, suddenly lucid, interjects and asks us to stop our "yackety-yakking." Responding immediately, as though seeing him for the first time, Keisha changes her tone and walks toward Mr. Jones, bends down to meet his line of vision, and assures him that everything is okay. Mr. Jones appears to relax in response to Keisha's attention. Keisha notices that Mr. Jones has soiled himself and asks Jodi to help her out. Together the two women pull Mr. Jones from his chair and walk him into the bathroom for a quick wash and change of clothes. Christina tells me there is little else she can do today and leads the way out of the apartment toward her county car.

On the Front Lines of Care

The story of Mr. Jones and Keisha is both touching and horrifying. The less-than-favorable conditions of Mr. Jones's care, his poverty, and the disarray of his living environment seem to confirm the sociological truism that social class and economic insecurity directly impact how one experiences aging and illness (Newman 1999a). Given this reality, it is tempting to place blame—for Mr. Jones's fall, for the condition of his home—at the feet of the person directly responsible for the day-to-day care of Mr. Jones: Keisha. Considering, however, that Keisha spends many unrecorded, uncompensated hours a week providing care to a relative stranger, both because there is no one else to do it and because Mr. Jones is too poor to receive more-comprehensive care (and perhaps also because she is unable to find a "better" job), it is fairer to say that Keisha is a critical resource for Mr. Jones rather than the primary threat to his safety or well-being. Recognizing, then, that both Mr. Jones and Keisha receive and give care, respectively, in conditions of poverty, with little support from family or health care providers, we can identify a set of broader social realities that inform their experiences.

Most obviously, the tenuous bond formed between Keisha and Mr. Jones reflects the many unanswered questions about long-term care in the United States. Why, for example, is Mr. Jones left unsupervised for hours at a time? Who pays for Mr. Jones's care, and why is he ineligible for more support? Why is Keisha doing this work? Is she qualified for the job? Does Mr. Jones have other options? Does Keisha?

In the ongoing policy conversations about long-term care in the United States, these broader questions take a backseat to the more immediate issues of supply and demand. In view of the projected growth in the number of senior citizens in the United States in the next ten to twenty years—the number of adults over sixty-five is expected to double by 2030—the question of how we will generate and sustain a "frontline" or direct-care workforce is of central concern (Institute of Medicine of the National Academies 2008). Often referred to as the "crisis in long-term care" or the "care gap" (Stone and Wiener 2001), the problem of finding sufficient numbers of quality care providers to meet the needs of the elderly is particularly acute in the United States, where family members are very often geographically dispersed and—even if they remain close by—struggle to care for a parent or loved one while also meeting the demands of career and children (Harrington Meyer 2000).

This crisis in care is expected to translate into an unprecedented growth in the personal home care industry, staffed by low-skilled paid caregivers such as certified nursing assistants (CNAs), home care aides and personal care assistants. The Bureau of Labor Statistics estimates that, between 1992 and 2005, home care aide was the second-fastest-growing occupation in the United States, with similar growth expected through 2016 (Bureau of Labor Statistics 2005; Paraprofessional Healthcare Institute 2008b; Smith and Baughman 2007b). If past conditions hold, most of the women—and a small number of men—who become home care aides will be unskilled, untrained, and underpaid (Crown, Ahlburg, and MacAdam 1995; Stone and Wiener 2001). In addition, paid caregiving is clearly a "racialized" occupation: poor women of color—often immigrants—are overrepresented in the population of home care aides and personal care assistants (Duffy 2007; Ehrenreich and Hochschild 2002; Harrington Meyer 2000; Nakano Glenn 1992).

Even with this anticipated growth in the home care industry, there remains a gap in knowledge about the challenges facing "frontline" workers (D. Stone 2000b; Wellin 2007). It is my intention in this book to enrich current debates over the long-term care crisis by describing in detail the constraints facing low-skilled caregivers on the front lines of care for the elderly and disabled, whose experiences are rendered invisible by a public that takes only passing interest in their work. Drawing on interviews with and observations of home care aides in California and Ohio, I describe the conditions under which low-skilled, low-waged caregivers provide for the needs of the elderly and chronically ill, paying particular attention to the material factors (namely, wages) and nonmaterial impulses (such as altruism, emotional attachment, and the drive for autonomy) that propel women into the job and sustain, or undermine, their occupational commitments.

Aides in the Home

The vast majority of care provided to the elderly, disabled, and chronically ill in the home is informal, assumed by family members who do not receive monetary compensation for their labor. Women traditionally bear the responsibility for unpaid caregiving, leading to near consensus in the literature that the social organization of care is an outgrowth of the emotional and occupational sexual division of labor (Cancian and Oliker 2001; Gordon, Benner, and Noddings 1996; Harrington Meyer 2000). Nearly 75 percent of people ages eighteen through sixty-four receiving long-term care assistance in the community (i.e., not in nursing homes) rely exclusively on unpaid caregivers, most of whom are women (Stone and Wiener 2001).

While it is crucial to recognize the work of informal caregivers, of increasing significance is the growing number of paid home care aides and nursing assistants who are filling in the care gap for families or individuals who cannot provide informal care due to realities of income, geography, or indifference (Harrington Meyer 2000; R. Stone 2001; Stone and Wiener 2001). When an elderly person or a family chooses home over institution, home care aides (also referred to as personal care assistants or chore workers) are often employed to share in hands-on or "direct" care. Such care includes feeding, bathing and tending to other aspects of personal hygiene, and providing companionship, activities known among long-term care professionals as activities of daily living, or ADLs. In recent years, concerns for patient safety, agency fears of liability, as well as state-level Nurse Practice Acts have limited the extent to which aides can provide even minor medical care, such as changing a dressing, administering insulin, or helping clients manage prescriptions (Reinhard 2001). In this climate, the work of the home care aide is largely relational in nature, meaning that the job requires a sustained and often reciprocal emotional connection to a client (Parks 2003). In short, home care work is as much emotional as it is physical.

Many aides serve as formal companions to their clients (as part of their job description) and also run errands and provide light housekeeping. Indeed, the range of work tasks associated with home care broadly mirrors the myriad tasks associated with the gendered division of labor in the home. In general, aides take on caregiving tasks that family members, specifically women in families, either cannot or will not do (Nakano Glenn 2000). Aides who do this work for pay often have many years of experience providing informal care to children and other family members without pay. Often called on in a family crisis, aides have caring trajectories that begin with unpaid care in their own home and then translate, usually in their middle years, to work as a paid caregiver. It is this history of informal caregiving that sets most aides on the path toward low-wage care work, reflecting an important link between a gendered division of labor in the home and the labor market.

Recent estimates (2006) suggest there are approximately eight hundred thousand home care aides employed in the United States, which is triple what the number was in 1989 (Kaye et al. 2006). The Bureau of Labor Statistics (2010) estimates that by 2018, there will be over 1 million home care aides in the United States. While aides in nursing homes and other institutional settings currently outnumber home care aides, the BLS projects that home care aides will outnumber their facility-based peers two to one within the next ten years (Paraprofessional Healthcare Institute 2008b). Some argue that the numbers are likely gross underestimates, as many home care workers and personal care assistants are self-employed or considered "independent providers," paid privately for their care and not easily tracked or counted (Institute of Medicine of the National Academies 2008). The more urgent problem suggested by the demographic data, however, is that the pressure for direct care workers, such as home care aides, continues to mount, even as demand for these workers outpaces the number of females projected to enter the labor force between 2006 and 2016 (Paraprofessional Healthcare Institute 2008b). Given this projected shortfall in labor supply, it is all the more urgent for the occupation of home care aide to become a quality job that will attract and retain low-skilled workers.

To date, there are few sociological studies on aides working in home settings, perhaps because work tasks and client-worker interactions unfold in a private context, making it difficult for researchers to render visible the labor associated with home care (Stone and Wiener 2001). Existing empirical investigations of aides tend to be descriptive in nature, with an emphasis on documenting the aggregate trends in the workforce, such as burnout, turnover, and average wages (Montgomery et al. 2005; Potter, Churilla, and Smith 2006; R. Stone 2004). Research to date shows that home care aides are, on average, poorly compensated and that the work is characterized by high rates of turnover and burnout (Brannon et al. 2002; Crown, Ahlburg, and MacAdam 1995; Stone and Wiener 2001).

The paucity of research on aides working in home settings stands in stark contrast to the sizable body of sociological research on nursing assistants and nursing aides who work in institutional settings (Chambliss 1996; Davies 1995; Diamond 1992; Foner 1994; Lopez 2006). Studies of aides in nursing homes—like Timothy Diamond's *Making Gray Gold* (1992) or Nancy Foner's *The Caregiving Dilemma* (1994)—identify the sources of stigma attached to low-level nursing work. They argue that the pressures to bureaucratize and "speed up" the caring process in nursing homes lead to poor living and working conditions for elderly residents and workers, respectively. While Foner disagrees somewhat with Diamond, arguing that commercialized, bureaucratic care can sometimes protect nursing home residents from aides who might act autonomously, both suggest that the general trend toward bureaucratic care and lack of worker autonomy harms residents and nursing aides alike.

Much of the social scientific literature on nursing aides focuses on this question of worker autonomy and the bureaucratization of care. However, once our focus shifts from institutional to home-based care, it is less clear how autonomy and bureaucratic control operate or whether they exist at all. Deborah Stone (2000a), in her study of home care, concludes that workers do in fact experience a conflict between bureaucratic rules and principles and their own ethic of care. Much like the health aides in Diamond's study, Stone found that home care workers went out of their way to spend extra time with clients and to pay out of their own pocket for client expenses, thereby preserving their own ethic of care. Stone suggests the crux of the problem is that "care in the public world is often incompatible with the norms, rules and expectations of care in the private world" (91), a situation particularly acute in home care where the private meanings associated with care are ever present.

Turning attention to paid care work in the home extends the literature on long-term care beyond the institution, allowing us to see how work constraints, such as the bureaucratization of care, vary when services are provided in an informal setting. Examining the work of nursing aides in the home also allows us to consider what happens when the boundaries between private and public space are blurred for both workers and their clients. Hochschild (2003) refers to this melding of work and family space as "marketized private life," where it is unclear which norms—familial, workplace, or both—guide social interaction. Home care is precisely such a site of marketized private life, where the "feeling rules" associated with aides' emotional labor dictate that care is both a familial obligation provided altruistically as well as a job that requires professionalism, objectivity, and distance. For this reason, home care is an ideal site of empirical investigation, especially when it comes to extending existing research on emotions and emotional labor at work.

Paid Care Work, Inequality, and Emotional Labor

Scholars of care work have long been interested in how women face both emotional and financial penalties for their paid care work (England, Budig, and Folbre 2002; Hochschild 1983). Women providing paid care—such as nannies, nurses, home care aides, and teachers—suffer a "wage penalty" for their work, relative to women and men in non–care work fields (England, Budig and Folbre 2002). Increasingly, paid caring labor is the work of women of color, who assume responsibility for caring work previously handled by unemployed white women in the home (Hondagneu-Sotelo 2001; Rollins 1985; Romero 1992). This racial division of paid reproductive labor (Nakano Glenn 1992) has "gone global," as women from developing countries migrate to the United States to work as nannies, domestics, or home care workers, often leaving their own children or elderly relatives at home and without care (Ehrenreich and Hochschild 2002; Parrenas 2001). In short, women who provide paid care to others often do so at great personal expense and with little financial reward.

The penalties of care work are due, in part, to the fact that women provide care within the less-than-favorable conditions of a service economy. Beyond the obvious material hardships that a service economy generates for low-skilled workers, students of care work also consider how service economies foster an "emotional proletariat" (Macdonald and Sirianni 1996), a sector of laborers for whom self-presentation and other personal characteristics become core job requirements. These relational work demands, what sociologists refer to as "emotional labor" (Hochschild 1983), can be detrimental to the worker because he or she experiences a "transmutation" of private feeling into a public display of emotion, resulting in alienation of self (Hochschild 1983, 19). Researchers offer examples of paid careworkers, such as nurses, who routinize care to manage their emotional labor (Chambliss 1996; Erickson and Grove 2007) or service workers who must evoke the feeling of care in a customer, so as to enhance the value of a material product, such as fast food or air travel (Hochschild 1983; Leidner 1993).

Given what we know about the demands of service work, care work in particular seems an obvious place to observe alienation that comes from emotional labor. The job requires, indeed demands, the performance of emotion to ensure the "product" of care is delivered. However, ample scholarship subsequent to Hochschild's *The Managed Heart* (1983) suggests that emotional labor does not have a uniformly negative impact on job satisfaction (Erickson and Grove 2008; Leidner 1993; Paules 1991; Wharton 1999; Wharton and Erickson 1993). One of the key conclusions to draw from the more recent work on emotional labor is that the consequences of emotional labor are largely dependent on the *context* of emotion management. Further, we now know that people, especially women, manage their emotional labor across multiple settings and roles (work and home; mother and employee) and that context matters for the overall impact of emotional labor on one's well-being and job satisfaction (Wharton 1993).

Care work generally, and home care specifically, provides an important point of discussion with respect to emotional labor. While the job demands "deep acting" on the part of the caregiver, I agree with Ashforth and Humphrey (1993) that the emotional labor of a home care worker is often born out of a long-term relationship with a client where genuine feelings of companionship emerge. Indeed, many caregivers emphasize the "fictive kinship" they have with clients, further complicating the nature of the emotional work (Karner 1998). Precisely because care work, including home care, involves long-term relationships between the caregiver and the recipient of care, Susan Himmelweit (1999) suggests that caring work is "incompletely commodified work," where both alienating and empowering forms of emotional labor exist. This supports Maria Ibarra's (2002) assertion that women caring for the elderly engage in authentic emotional labor, distinguishing them from what are characterized as emotional proletarians. Of course, the existence of authentic emotion in care work does not preclude the alienation of the self that Hochschild predicts, but the unique context of both care and service work make home care work a rich site from which to examine new terrain in the ongoing study of emotional labor.

For aides working in the home, the boundaries of work/home and public/private space are fundamentally blurred, which in turn shapes the way in which aides provide and interpret their care. On the one hand, aides are paid employees who must follow procedures and regulations as they strive to meet client needs. On the other hand, caregiving in the space of a home cues aides and clients to a less formal set of interactional rules, akin to family relationships rather than those associated with work. In this context, the motivation for providing care also becomes confused as aides (and clients) wonder whether care is provided for the sake of love or money. Most caregivers are likely motivated by emotional connections to clients and their need for pay, but as Viviana Zelizer (2005) points out, we live in a society that believes that love and money are incompatible "hostile worlds" that should remain eternally separate (lest we sully the altruistic dimensions of love). Walking the "love or money" line is particularly cruel for home care aides, who commit themselves both physically and emotionally to clients for a paltry minimum wage. Despite the obvious inequality embedded within this exchange, most aides choose to emphasize the relational aspects of their work and downplay their own pecuniary interests, thereby reinforcing the idea that love and money are irreconcilable.

As aides cultivate companionship with clients, confusion over home/work and love/money is exacerbated. The ability to form genuine ties to clients is a source of pride for aides who view it as a form of skilled, emotional labor that gives their work lives meaning and improves quality of life for clients. At the same time, companionship can complicate formal work arrangements between aides and clients, sometimes resulting in the overwork or emotional overinvestment of caregivers who find it difficult to extract themselves from clients who feel and act more like friends or family than employers. Labor advocates are quick to point out that focusing on companionship also obscures the formal, physical labor associated with caregiving and makes it difficult for aides to mount legitimate claims to fair wages and labor protections. Aides (and some of their clients) may view companionship as work, but the law unfortunately does not recognize it as such.[2]

Despite compelling claims that aides are "more than companions," I suggest that the relationship between aide and client—and the related "input" of emotional labor—is central to understanding the work of aides. This relational work of companionship (Parks 2003) influences workers' job satisfaction and their emotional health, as well as their identities and sense of self, in ways that are not always predictable or obvious. *The Caring Self* explores both the positive and negative consequences of emotional labor for worker subjectivity, arguing that aides actively construct and narrate a sense of self, what I call the caring self, by drawing directly (and strategically) on the relational dimensions of their work.

Investigating the link between emotional labor and identity at work is crucial if we are to understand the factors that lead to high rates of worker turnover and burnout. I contend that current discussions about long-term care either ignore the emotional labor associated with low-skilled care work, or assume—with little empirical evidence—that emotional labor has only deleterious consequences for caregivers (Erickson and Grove 2008; Lopez 2006; Nakano Glenn 1992). In view of concerns about the recruitment and retention of frontline workers, it makes sense to carefully interrogate the reasons—including affective reasons—why women and some men become paid caregivers and why they stay on (or leave) the job. While by no means a treatise on workforce policy, this book aims to insert the voices and experiences of frontline workers into current discussions about the crisis in long-term care.

The Rewards of Emotional Labor: Rosa's Story

Rosa is a fifty-year-old Latina who migrated to the United States from Guatemala with her husband in the early 1990s so that he could pursue a doctoral degree in California. After having an affair with a woman in his department, Rosa's husband moved out, leaving Rosa to care for her son and unborn child. Rosa immediately took a job cleaning office buildings, but determined quickly that she could not make a living from the wages, two hundred dollars a week for over forty hours of work. While looking for employment, Rosa went into labor with her second child and ended up in the emergency room, where she waited in a hallway for hours before being roomed. Although terrified—Rosa's English at the time was quite limited—the birth itself was transformative for Rosa. She recalled the kindness of a nursing aide who helped her immediately after the delivery: "This lady came, she took care of me, she cleaned me up....I will never forget those hands. That changed my life...those hands were so special to me. So I wanted to care for somebody, too."

Rosa found a job in a nursing home as an aide after giving birth to her son, but she became disillusioned after experiencing heavy patient load, long hours, and what she perceived to be poor-quality care for patients. Eventually, Rosa found work as a home care aide for an Alzheimer's patient in his seventies who had a drinking problem. Rosa enjoyed working with her client and drove him each day to feed the birds, coaxing him with the refrain, "Bread, not beer." She soon learned she had a talent for elder care and took on a number of clients with dementia. Rosa believed, as she still does today, that it is her job to "work the cells of the [clients'] brains" by taking them to places where they are "stimulated." Rosa told of her outings to the beach with a male client with dementia:

> I took him to smell the ocean, to smell the water in the ocean and touch...the sand. And walk without shoes in the sand, and other kinds of things. Going to the mountain and watching all the kinds of trees, what kind of wood the trees are. That's the kind of work I like, but there's not [much] work like that.

Rosa developed a strong bond with this client and, years later, still receives regular letters and phone calls from his family. The day I interviewed Rosa in her home, for example, she played back a phone message from the client that she had saved on her answering machine as a keepsake. The message was warm and familial in tone, as the client spoke of missing Rosa and feeling that "the house was sad" without her.

Rosa's love of and commitment to her clients does not mean her work life is free of adversity. She has clients who treat her poorly, and she often works in conditions that are unhealthy both physically and emotionally (one of her clients is a "hoarder," for example, so Rosa must work around the detritus in the house and put up with whatever toxins she suspects are lurking under the mess). Rosa also struggles to pay the rent, has no health insurance, and relies on her son, a junior in college, to help her out when money is tight. Rosa has worked as a maid and resents the fact that you can make more money caring for the objects in someone's home than you can caring for an elderly or disabled person living in that home.

Even with these hardships and frustrations, Rosa's story is a poignant case of an aide who emotionally invests in her clients' physical and emotional health and then experiences a sense of emotional well-being and job satisfaction as a result of her labor. While the details of Rosa's experiences are indeed unique (few caregivers take their clients on sensory excursions), the intensity of her bond with a client was echoed by many of the caregivers interviewed. More often than not, workers report strong emotional ties to clients, even when working conditions are otherwise adverse (low wages, no benefits, erratic work schedules, lack of training). Rosa, and other workers like her, illustrate that while aides often experience inequality on the job, there are other aspects of the work from which they draw meaning and satisfaction. In short, aides' accounts prompt us to consider circumstances when emotional exploitation does not necessarily follow from material exploitation. This is not to downplay the nature or consequences of inequality for caregivers. Rather, exploring the affective and emotional ties aides form with clients allows us to understand how workers interpret and maneuver within a job that is low paying, low prestige and often unpredictable.

Researching Home Care

The idea for this book was formed in my apartment, around a dining room table. While in graduate school, I often had informal dinners and gatherings with my nonsociology friends who had "real" jobs as public servants, educators, or social workers. Conversations ranged from politics and relationships to daily dramas at work. Friends employed as caseworkers by In-Home Supportive Services (IHSS) in Central City, California, would regularly hold court with their compelling, sometimes funny, tales about elderly clients and their paid caregivers.

One evening, I found myself drawn into a story about a frail elderly woman who lived around the corner from me in a low-income housing unit. I had passed this building hundreds of times, unaware that she and nearly one hundred other poor, elderly residents populated the complex (a drab structure with an institutional feel, replete with overgrown shrubs and a concrete facade). Perhaps it was the fact that this elderly woman, Ruth, lived close by, or perhaps it was the details of her circumstances that captured my attention (such as her tendency to use a rusty old shopping cart for support as she maneuvered within her three-hundred-square-foot apartment). Either way, I wanted to know more. As a medical sociologist interested in issues of aging and inequality, I felt an urgency to under-stand how Ruth and other low-income elderly or chronically ill people get through the day in a city that renders them invisible. My interest, at least initially, was in the people needing care, not the aides who provide it.

With more than a little help from my friends, I arranged meetings with managers and administrators at IHSS, a state-funded program that provides custodial care (cleaning, cooking, bathing, etc.) to elderly and disabled individuals who qualify on the basis of income. I did my best to convince various gatekeepers that further sociological attention should be paid to the unmet needs of poor elders, and most (although not all) agreed. After countless phone calls, two Institutional Review Board approval pro-cesses, and a few delays, I was given permission to accompany IHSS so-cial workers and public health nurses on "ride arounds" to client homes. Elated, I knew that I had found a way to meet and learn about the Ruths of the world.

Not long after I gained access to IHSS, I traveled with my social-worker friend to Ruth's apartment. As we took the elevator to the seventh floor, I prepared myself to meet a frail, older white woman debilitated by rheumatoid arthritis and in desperate need of support. The person I first encountered, however, was not Ruth. It was Annie, Ruth's paid caregiver, a very large African American woman in her midforties. Annie greeted us politely and escorted us down the hall to the apartment, saying very little but smiling. As we entered the apartment, I could hear Ruth calling to Annie with some urgency; she needed help getting to the bathroom.

After introducing myself and explaining my purpose for being there, I crouched in the corner and observed as Ruth and Annie moved through their routines and my friend (the social worker) ran through a list of ques-tions. Ruth was as frail as I had expected, but her acerbic tongue (mostly directed at Annie) distracted me from her condition. I became intrigued by the relationship between these two women. It was clear that Ruth was capable of doing very little without Annie's help and that the apartment, spotless and uncluttered, was maintained on a daily basis by the aide. Annie explained that she spent hours every day keeping the environment clean, free of dirt or chemicals that might irritate Ruth's sensitive system. Each morning when Annie arrived, the women made their way to the bathroom, where Annie washed Ruth's hair and shaved her legs. Ruth could not tolerate any amount of stubble on her legs, so this ritual was never skipped. Annie told my friend that Ruth had become incontinent and that they did not have a regular supply of pads since Medicare won't reimburse arthritis patients for incontinence supplies. The few remaining pads left in the apartment came from a visiting nurse and from Annie, who purchased a pack at her own expense. We learned that Ruth was also refusing to see her physical therapist when he made house calls, so Annie did her best to "work" Ruth's muscles on a daily basis. Annie had a quiet confidence about her, and seemed able to ignore Ruth's insults and jabs. I later learned that Annie had been with Ruth longer than any other caregiver, and that most aides in the past had left on account of Ruth's demanding nature and the delusions she experiences as a result of one of her medications. (Ruth had coaxed her last aide to drive twenty miles into the suburbs to visit her son, only to admit on arrival that no such son existed.)

I left this visit with a new set of questions. Why did Annie do this work? Was she paid enough? What did she like (if anything) about her work? Did she consider Ruth a friend or a client? How did Ruth feel about Annie? I certainly remained interested in documenting the needs of low-income elders, but I quickly realized that any story about long-term care must also be a story about the aides working on the front lines. I switched gears and began to concentrate on the relationships that form between aides and clients, with primary focus on the aide side of the dyad. From what I could tell, these paid caregivers had been rather neglected and rendered even more invisible than the elders for whom they labor.

Focusing on the work experiences of home care aides proved somewhat difficult initially, since they work in private homes, out of public view, and congregate together on an irregular basis (if at all). I managed to recruit a few aides during ride arounds with nurses and social workers, but this strategy did not readily yield respondents. I began to frequent training sessions, union meetings, and social gatherings, introducing myself as a sociologist interested in the work of home care aides. I also started talking to the owner of a private agency—It's For You—who granted me permission to recruit workers from her staff roster. Between the IHSS meetings and the private agency, I found a considerable number of aides willing to talk to me. Later, after I moved to Ohio for my first academic job, I interviewed aides living in the small city of Middletown who worked for an agency called Maximum Care.

In all, I conducted formal interviews with thirty-three home care workers (mostly women, although five men were interviewed) and observed and interacted with hundreds others, either while they worked in client homes or during various trainings and meetings. I learned quickly that aides aren't paid very much considering the emotional and physical labor associated with the job—on average about nine dollars an hour in California

TABLE 1. Age, Race, and Employer of Home Care Aides Interviewed (N = 33)

Name (pseudonym)	Age	Race	Employer
Andrew	53	African American	IHSS
Jennifer	54	White	IHSS
José	53	Latino	IHSS
Joyce	71	African American	IHSS
Karen	47	White	IHSS
Kelly	60	White	IHSS
Lete	36	Latino	IHSS
Mark	44	Asian American	IHSS
Martina	57	African American	IHSS
Maureen	68	White	IHSS
Michael	33	Asian American	IHSS
Rosa	50	Latino	IHSS
Sally	52	African American	IHSS
Camilla	39	African American	It's For You
Fahima	49	Latino	It's For You
George	33	Asian	It's For You
Hannah	33	Asian	It's For You
Isabel	38	Latino	It's For You
Jackie	42	African American	It's For You
Katy	65	Asian American	It's For You
Meghan	28	White	It's For You
Sandra	47	White	It's For You
Sophie	48	White	It's For You
Dawn	38	White	Maximum Care
Dot	51	White	Maximum Care
Kristen	65	White	Maximum Care
Maggie	62	White	Maximum Care
Mary	67	White	Maximum Care
Patty	35	White	Maximum Care
Shelly	28	White	Maximum Care
Tammy	51	White	Maximum Care
Tiffany	48	White	Maximum Care
Virginia	62	White	Maximum Care

and eight dollars an hour in Ohio (Paraprofessional Healthcare Institute 2008c). Most have no formal health care skills or training, although a handful of the aides I talked to are licensed certified nursing assistants, or CNAs. Aides come from all racial and ethnic backgrounds, but there is a disproportionate number of black and Latino workers in the field, especially in states such as California and New York (Smith and Baughman 2007a). The recipients of care—the "clients"—also come from all walks of life. Some are poor and receive care via government entitlement, while others pay some or all of the cost associated with their care. In terms of race and ethnicity, the clients are as diverse as the aides who care for them.

As I pulled together these early observations, it became clear to me that home care aides work in a demanding service job characterized by limited mobility, substandard wages and benefits, and few labor protections. For these reasons alone, I wanted to document and share their stories. As I continued talking to aides, however, I realized that they didn't always define their work as limiting or "dead end." Most acknowledged the low pay and lack of benefits but were also quick to emphasize the rewards that come from the affective dimensions of care, such as cultivating companionship with clients or developing ties with families. Some even talked about leaving other service jobs in search of home care precisely because it gave them an opportunity to interact with others in a meaningful way. Rather than view this as a form of false consciousness, I sought to understand how the relational aspects of home care serve as a positive source of identity for aides, while at the same time being attentive to the possibility that emotional ties are also stressful for workers. With these central questions in mind, I set out to document the experiences of home care aides, in the hope of explaining how they find dignity, purpose, and meaning in a job with very few extrinsic rewards.

Explanation of Terms

A number of terms specific to long-term care are used in this book. To avoid any confusion that might come from the discrepancy between common and professional use of terms, I briefly define here the most important and/or confusing terms found in the book. The most general term used in the discussion is "long-term care," which refers to nonacute care offered either in institutions (such as nursing homes) or in the home. Within the broad category of long-term care, I distinguish between two types of care: "informal" and "formal." Informal care refers to the unpaid care provided to family members and friends, generally in the home. Formal care, in contrast, is the paid work of nurses, doctors, or nursing aides that takes place in either a home or an institutional setting. As the book illustrates, however, the line between formal and informal care is not always clearly delineated in the lives of many caregivers since the vast majority of aides juggle both formal and informal caregiving responsibilities (caring for a child or elderly parent at home, for example, and then offering paid services to a client outside the home).

In the pages that follow, I also use the term "custodial care" to refer to the work of home care aides. Custodial care refers to the provision of nonmedical care—including cooking, cleaning, and bathing—usually relegated to unskilled health aides or attendants. Home care workers are minimally trained and are prohibited from administering medication, cleaning wounds, or changing catheters, among other tasks. Given this restriction, many aides refer to their work as "companion care," emphasizing the interactive, relational work that occupies much of their time.

There is little consensus on what to call workers who provide unskilled home care. I label these caregivers "home care workers" or "home care aides," since these terms are commonly used by workers themselves. Organizations that advocate on behalf of aides generally refer to the population as "personal and home care workers," but few aides use this terminology.[3] It should be noted that home care aides are generally not home *health* aides. Home care aides provide longer-term, custodial care of clients, whereas home health aides (not discussed in this book) care for patients who have recently been released from the hospital and who need short-term (lasting a few days or up to six weeks) postoperative or postacute care. Home care aides generally work independently or as part of a team of aides when caring for a patient; home health aides are usually under the direct supervision of a registered nurse (RN) who is responsible for coordinating patient care.[4]

Organization of the Book

This book is organized around two interrelated themes: the way in which paid home care structurally disadvantages low-wage women, while at the same time it personally fortifies many who derive value from their emotional connections to elderly and disabled clients. How aides find meaning and identity at work—what I call the caring self—within the very real context of structural disadvantage (poverty, speedup of work, low wages, few benefits) is the central question of the book. Elaborating on this tension between occupational inequality and identity formation at work, the first half of the book documents the many constraints facing home care aides, including the realities of poverty, injury, and workplace exploitation. The second half of the book focuses on aides' construction of the caring self at work and the implications of this identity formation for caregivers' job satisfaction and self-advocacy.

In chapter 1, I begin the discussion of inequality in home care, introducing the reader to the political, economic, and biographical factors that propel women into paid caregiving. Similar to domestics and nannies, home care aides often find themselves doing care work for a wage simply because the job is one of few available in the service sector. Once on the job, aides find themselves contending with the "speedup" of work, the piecemeal nature of employment (i.e., working part-time for multiple clients), low wages, and poor benefits. These macrostructural constraints intersect with the social locations of the workers themselves, many of whom are poor, without formal education or job training, or otherwise disenfranchised due to their race, class, or immigrant status. Certainly all women, irrespective of race and class, suffer penalties—both social and financial—for assuming roles as caregivers (England, Budig, and Folbre 2002). The chapter makes the case that caregiving penalties are more severe for home care aides and other low-skilled careworkers since they provide both unpaid and paid care within the context of significant economic insecurity.

Chapter 1 goes on to consider how the biographies and "career lines" (Spenner, Otto, and Call 1982) of home care aides also bear the markings of structural inequality, especially in relation to aides' personal histories as informal caregivers in their own families. I dub these life patterns "caring trajectories," which begin with the unpaid care of a family member, friend, or neighbor and lead, ultimately, to employment in paid caregiving. Aides who follow this trajectory (nearly the entire sample) cite "natural" caregiving abilities as the primary reason they end up assuming responsibility for both child care and elder care in their own families, and why they find themselves in paid care work. Worker beliefs in an essential disposition to care is a key component of the caring self, and reflects a certain internalization of long-standing gender norms that dictate care as "women's work" (Cancian and Oliker 2001). Aides' convictions about their "natural" caregiving abilities obscure what is in fact a lifetime of "constrained choices" with respect to caregiving obligations (Bird and Rieker 2008). Even so, years of informal caregiving do supply aides with a degree of "emotional capital" (Cahill 1999; Reay 2004), a relational skill set that translates into a sense of confidence, ability, and "giftedness" when it comes to caregiving. Although aides' emotional capital holds clear occupational value, at least for workers and clients, it does not hold much social value, given society's tendency to devalue nurturant skills and care work more generally (Cancian and Oliker 2001). As such, aides' emotional capital is an important foundation for the caring self but does little to ameliorate the larger structural inequalities associated with paid caregiving.

Chapter 2, "Doing the Dirty Work," describes in ethnographic detail the nature and intensity (both physical and emotional) of direct care of the elderly and disabled, exploring the constraints facing aides who provide direct care. Certain conditions of work—such as financial insecurity, on-the-job injury, lack of training, and bureaucratic constraints on care—produce distress and fatigue for home care aides. With respect to emotional labor, the chapter establishes that there are times when aides' emotional ties to clients prove overwhelming and lead to feelings of burnout, exhaustion, fatigue, and a sense of alienation. Providing companionship around the clock for clients who are often lonely or depressed can take a psychological toll on workers, for example. Aides also find themselves providing "surplus care," working additional hours without compensation or offering to do tasks outside their scope of work, simply because there is no one else to do it. In these moments, broader institutional and organizational realities directly impact the way in which aides experience their emotional labor. These factors reinforce the inequality associated with paid care work, with potential consequences for worker satisfaction and burnout.

It is at this juncture in the book that I turn to consider the affective rewards and identity-affirming aspects of home care. Aides report actively pursuing a career in home care precisely because the work is conducive to forming relational ties with clients, something that is unavailable to them in other caregiving and service jobs. Chapter 3, "The Rewards of Caring," suggests that aides find a degree of functional and relational autonomy in home care that allows them to engage in emotional labor "on their own terms." Aides also find dignity in the fictive kinship bonds formed with clients and their families, a factor that works in tandem with autonomy to lay the foundation for the caring self. As a "situated identity," the caring self is multifaceted and formed in the context of aides' interaction with clients, other caregivers, and other health care professionals. Aides construct the caring self by engaging in three types of "identity talk" (Snow and Anderson 1987): professing care as natural and innate, emphasizing service to others, and marking boundaries between themselves and "uncaring" others. In the formation of the caring self, it is clear that *talking* about emotional labor is as important as the experience of emotional labor itself (at least to the aide), since communicating and performing emotionality helps reify the caring self in the eyes of clients and others. As such, *talk* of companionship and ties to clients operates as an interactional strategy that aides use to reassert skill, reinforce their social value, and assert an authentic self.

Chapter 3 also makes the case that social locations of race, class, and gender are crucial to the development of the caring self. While feminist sociologists have long argued that race, nationality, class, and gender all influence the odds that one will become a low-wage caregiver (Duffy 2007; Nakano Glenn 1992), little research addresses how these social locations shape the way in which workers do the job or feel about the work. The chapter attempts to address this gap by teasing out the links between social location, emotional labor, and worker identity. What becomes clear is that for aides of color, particularly African American aides, experiences of discrimination on the job (usually from clients) profoundly affect the way these workers experience the caring self and narrate their care. Non-native-born aides from Mexico, the Philippines, and Latin America experience their care slightly differently and make the case that they possess superior caregiving skills due to their racial or ethnic backgrounds. Rather than viewing these differences as somehow essential or part of individual- or group-level disposition, the chapter concludes that all aides construct a caring self on the job, but that this identity varies by social location in notable ways.

While chapters 1 through 3 explore the tension between inequality and identity in care work, chapter 4, "Organizing Home Care," explores the question of worker advocacy, specifically unionization. Organizing campaigns in California and Ohio are considered, with particular attention paid to the way that rights-based organizing frames in California coalesce (and sometimes collide) with components of the caring self, namely, themes of family and service. Drawing on aides' views and perceptions of unions, the chapter discusses how future organizing efforts might recognize the importance of the caring self for worker dignity and job satisfaction.

The conclusion brings together central claims about identity and inequality in home care and suggests ways that the empirical findings about aides' work experiences might enrich ongoing discussions about maintaining a robust direct care workforce. As aides tell us, there are both constraints and rewards to home care work, especially when it comes to the emotional or relational aspects of the job. I summarize ways that the caring self reinforces aides' commitments to their clients, at the same time that it essentializes women's roles as "natural" caregivers and obscures home care as a form of *waged* labor. I conclude the book with a discussion of policy changes that would improve working conditions for aides and ensure higher quality of care for clients. Specifically, I discuss in detail the "companionship exemption" of the Fair Labor Standards Act, which excludes personal and home care aides from wage and overtime protections, largely due to the informal nature of the work they provide. I suggest that reforms to the FLSA must be accompanied by empirically grounded and theoretically engaged discussions of the meaning of companionship, so that fair value is given to the emotional and relational work of caregiving.

The Costs of Caring

LETE

Lete came to the United States in 1992 from Sinaloa, Mexico, at the age of twenty-six, to join her sister and aunt living in California. Soon after emigrating, Lete found herself caring for her aunt, who had fallen ill with a terminal form of cancer. In addition to providing care at home, Lete secured a part-time job in a factory at night, assembling computers for $9.50 an hour. Lete eventually earned her GED from a local community college and then enrolled in a few night courses—mostly nursing and computer science related—to try to identify a new career path. After her aunt died, Lete decided she could no longer justify the expense of community college, so she quit to find full-time work. She secured a job as a packer in the warehouse of a big-box chain store, making fourteen dollars an hour with health benefits.

Several months into her packing job, Lete heard through a friend that IHSS was hiring home care aides with no training required. Within a matter of days, Lete was assigned to work with a frail ninety-two-year-old white woman, Mavis, who lived alone and required help with bathing, dressing, cleaning, and cooking. Although Lete made decent money working the night shift at the warehouse, she felt drawn to Mavis. Having "prayed for a purpose" on her arrival to the United States, Lete believed God led her to caregiving, first for her aunt and now for Mavis. She took the job with Mavis but continued to work nights at the warehouse, in need of the higher wages and health benefits offered with the packing job.

Mavis proved to be a demanding and difficult woman to care for—insulting Lete for being overweight and accusing her of theft, for example—but Lete feels they now have a close bond. Lete wants to work full-time caring for Mavis, but such a change would require her to leave the night shift at the warehouse, which pays six dollars an hour more and offers insurance. Between the two jobs, Lete works nearly seventy hours a week. She says that the hours are required to ensure that she can pay her rent and send small sums of money back to family in Mexico. Even though Lete essentially works around the clock to make ends meet, she still takes care of Mavis on Saturday "for free." Lete feels Mavis needs the care and it is her "calling" to do so, saying that "caregiving is what God has put me on this earth to do."

Lete comes from a family with a strong commitment to the care of elders, and she spent time as a young adult caring for her grandfather, alongside her mother and other sisters. Lete's sister, Alicia, works as a child care provider and hopes to open her own day care; Lete describes her sister as "another me," referring to their shared proclivities for caregiving. Lete tells me that her talent for caregiving comes, in part, from spending her formative years in Mexico. She contrasts Mexico with the United States with respect to the care of elders and says that "[U.S.] culture lacks an interest in elders . . . young people don't think they are important." She adds, "We don't appreciate what they've done . . . we are losing what's important in life, values." When I ask Lete to compare her caregiving job to her work in the warehouse, she tells me that the caregiving job is harder because there "[you] feel pressure, because you don't know how she [Mavis] is going to be." This work is more difficult, she tells me, than trying to meet the piece rate in her eight-hour shift at the warehouse. Even so, Lete would leave the packing job if, as she put it, "the money weren't so bad" in caregiving.

Providing Care in the Context of Poverty

As Lete's story illustrates, many nursing aides provide ongoing care to others in the context of serious economic hardship. The job of home care aide (or any direct care worker for that matter) is an entry-level health care occupation that requires little formal education, offers minimal training, and generally carries very little promise of vertical mobility (Crown, Ahlburg, and MacAdam 1995; Stone and Wiener 2001; Yamada 2002). As such, nursing aides, whether they work in a private home or a facility, are part of the very same low-wage service sector that has become the focus of attention for a growing number of sociologists of inequality (Edin and Lein 1997; Leidner 1993; Munger 2002; Sherman 2007).

Home care is a growth industry, especially in the areas of personal care and homemaker services (Paraprofessional Healthcare Institute 2008b; Stone and Wiener 2001). Unlike institutional care (i.e., nursing home or convalescent care), home care is a largely unregulated industry composed of a complex array of publicly funded and proprietary agencies (Benjamin 1993; Stone and Wiener 2001). Some aides work for private, for-profit agencies (such as It's For You or Maximum Care), while others work for state agencies like IHSS, under what is called a "consumer-directed" model. In such a model, clients theoretically hire, train, supervise, and fire aides, while the organization overseeing care (e.g., IHSS) administers payment to workers. In consumer-directed care, agencies label aides "independent providers," a misnomer that allows the state to distance itself—at least in name—from the responsibilities and liabilities that agency employers face in the private sector. Certainly for aides in the field, the distinction drawn between consumer-directed and agency-based care is overstated, since in either context workers provide care to clients and are paid a wage by a third party (either an agency or state entity).

In California and Ohio, few agencies require advance training of aides (and minimal on-the-job training), although some agencies mandate CPR certification and evidence of basic first aid skills. There is also evidence that the scope of work radically varies from state to state, from agency to agency, and even from client to client, depending on whether that client's care is paid for by public monies or private insurance (Institute of Medicine of the National Academies 2008). In real terms, this means that an aide working multiple jobs, which is often the case, can go from being a "housecleaner" in one context, to changing bandages or Foley catheters in another. Many of the aides interviewed expressed frustration that job descriptions and scope of work change so radically by agency, with often no obvious rationale for the discrepancy.

With respect to pay and benefits there is little standardization, but successful organizing campaigns in California, New York, and Oregon represent an important shift in the bargaining power of home care workers in the United States (Mareschal 2006, 2007). In Northern California in 2004, average wages for an IHSS worker after unionization rose to ten dollars an hour, from the minimum wage of only seven dollars a few years earlier (Howes 2006). Bracketing the issue of unionization, and taking real wages into account, a bleaker picture emerges. In 2006, the real median hourly wage for personal and home care workers was $7.96 in California, and $7.40 in Ohio. These numbers are slightly higher than the national average real wage for aides of $7.17. The more distressing reality is that real wages for aides have actually declined, from $7.50 in 1999 to $7.14 in 2006. Geographic variation is apparent as well. In 2006, Texas reported a real wage of $5.41 for aides, while in the same year real wages in Alaska were $11.38 (Paraprofessional Healthcare Institute 2008c). Whether an aide can garner a living wage from home care appears highly dependent on geographic location and the extent to which the labor force is organized. One thing is certain: higher wages positively impact worker turnover (Howes 2006), which suggests that the material inequality associated with direct care is a considerable constraint for aides. Ample evidence now exists to support the claim that raising wages would indeed help address the perennial problem of workforce turnover (Howes 2006; Kemper et al. 2008).

Addressing turnover, however, is no small task, as rates of attrition are high for personal and home care aides, as well as for aides working in nursing homes. Estimates of turnover range between 45 and 100 percent for the general population of direct care workers, depending on study sample size and different formulas for calculating turnover (Ejaz et al. 2008; Harris-Kojetin et al. 2004). A majority of aides working for IHSS, the largest employer of home care aides in California, leave the job within three years

(Benjamin, Matthias, and Franke 2000). While turnover is the scourge of the industry, resulting in annual losses totaling over $2 billion (Ejaz et al. 2008; Seavey 2004), the constant hemorrhaging of caregivers also reflects uncertainties *workers* face as they traverse service jobs in the new economy (V. Smith 2001). As the accounts of workers in this book demonstrate, aides move in and out of home care work—sometimes for personal reasons, often for financial reasons—but tend to return because there are few other options available to them. This movement in and out of care work, while common, takes a toll on workers who wish for a more predictable occupational path.

Beyond poor wages, there are many reasons why turnover is so high among nursing aides, including lack of benefits, insufficient training, workload stressors, and the high emotional demands of the work (Brannon et al. 2002). As the women and men in this book attest, health, sick leave, and retirement benefits are generally unavailable to them, although organized workers usually have better access to benefits beyond wages (Howes 2004). It is a cruel reality that many aides, who spend their days tending to the health care needs of others, go without care themselves, sometimes for the duration of their careers. Many of the "veterans" interviewed for this study, some with job experience that exceeds fifteen years, have never had health insurance. When asked what they do when they get sick, almost all responded with the eerie refrain, "I don't get sick."[1] Data on the insurance status of direct care workers supports this anecdotal evidence. In fact, advocates for the direct care workforce refer to the insurance crisis among aides as the "invisible care gap," worthy of the same kind of attention (and investment of resources) as the care gap confronting the elderly (Paraprofessional Healthcare Institute 2008a). Estimates published in 2008 suggest that nearly 30 percent of direct care workers in the United States lack health coverage, making them twice as likely as the general public to go without insurance (Paraprofessional Healthcare Institute 2008a). Among the ten aides I interviewed in Ohio, only two of the women have health insurance (through their partners); among the California aides, one-third of the twenty-three aides have insurance. Aides working for It's For You and Maximum Care were the least likely to have insurance, whereas aides working for IHSS were more likely to be insured, due in part to the successful organizing campaign of publicly employed aides in California (Boris and Klein 2006; Delp and Quan 2002; Howes 2004).

While there are very few formal job requirements for nursing aides, working as a paid caregiver to an elderly or disabled person does necessitate a set of informal skills, including emotional intelligence, physical strength, and work flexibility. Aides receive very little training from agencies to help foster these skills, although, now organized, IHSS workers are offered regular, voluntary training sessions on a range of topics. Some home care aides begin their careers as certified nursing assistants (CNAs) or state tested nursing assistants (STNAs). Among the workers interviewed, however, only those who work simultaneously in nursing facilities and home care renew their license each year (most nursing homes now require CNA or STNA certification). While half of the aides began with a license, only five renew annually. This is not surprising given that the difference in pay between a certified aide and a noncertified aide is usually negligible. Predictably, poor training seems to go hand in hand with lack of career advancement: a statewide study in California found that only 5 to 12 percent of IHSS workers experience vertical mobility and go on to train as a licensed vocational nurse (LVN), arguably the next step on the career ladder (Ong et al. 2002).

Inadequate training and poor job mobility, combined with low wages and high turnover, mean that aides who find themselves in this line of work tend to face ongoing economic uncertainty. A majority of aides in the sample described working multiple jobs for multiple clients to ensure enough weekly income to simply pay their own bills and housing costs. While I did not ask respondents to reveal their monthly gross income, aides talked at length about relying on public assistance for health care and, occasionally, for food (i.e., food stamps). Nine of the aides interviewed have one or more children under the age of eighteen. The sample roughly mirrors national trends that suggest 40 percent of home care workers have a child under the age of eighteen and must therefore juggle paid and unpaid caregiving responsibilities (Smith and Baughman 2007a; D. Stone 2000b). Wages for home care workers in California and Ohio range between eight and ten dollars per hour and hardly constitute a living wage, especially in situations where the caregiver is a single parent, which is true for roughly 22 percent of home care aides nationally (Smith and Baughman 2007a). Although some economists argue that recent improvements in wages and benefits make home care a "good" job financially (Howes 2006), the individual aides in this study would beg to differ. Respondents, especially those with dependent children, report that they often work multiple jobs or their kids "go without" from time to time because the wages, although a drastic improvement from the minimum wage of a few years ago, are inadequate to sustain a family.

It is not surprising, given these working conditions, to learn that three in ten direct care workers live in households that have poverty or near-poverty income levels (Paraprofessional Healthcare Institute 2008a). In California, 25 percent of all IHSS caregivers received welfare at some point between 1995 and 2000 (Ong et al. 2002). The number dropped to 10 per-cent in 2000, but it is not clear whether this reflects successful transition to full-time employment and the benefits of increased wages or if this drop in the welfare rolls reflects the simple fact that many Temporary Assistance to Needy Families (TANF) recipients have "timed out" of income support and are no longer counted on the welfare rolls.

It is important to keep in mind that aides are not the only social actors grappling with poverty in this story. In both Ohio and California, Medicaid waiver programs allow low-income residents to opt for state-subsidized personal care in lieu of institutional care.[2] As a result, most agencies cater to both privately and publicly insured clients. With the exception of one aide, each caregiver introduced in the book serves at least one low-income person (some care exclusively for low-income clients). As we will see in subsequent chapters, when both sides of the caring dyad are poor, aides are sometimes quick to overextend themselves both emotionally and finan-cially to clients with whom they share similar conditions of poverty.

Racial Formations in Direct Care Work

It is clear from the above discussion that the working poor—those with low socioeconomic status (SES)—provide the bulk of low-skilled care to the elderly and disabled in the United States. Taking an even closer look at the demographic profile of workers, we see that race and ethnicity fur-ther compound the link between paid care work and social inequality. In the words of Evelyn Nakano Glenn (1992), there is a clear "racial divi-sion of paid reproductive labor" associated with personal and home care work, meaning that women of color are overrepresented in occupations like nanny, maid, and home care worker. Nearly half of all home care aides

nationally are white women, but black women and Latinas are disproportionately represented in the occupation, representing 24 percent and
21 percent of the workforce respectively (Smith and Baughman 2007a).
Of all home care aides, 22 percent are foreign-born, further evidence that
the world is witnessing a transfer of caring labor from the global South to
the global North (Ehrenreich and Hochschild 2002; Smith and Baughman
2007a). Direct care, not surprisingly, is female dominated: 89 percent of the
workforce are women (Smith and Baughman 2007a). To the extent that
men enter the occupation, it is men of color who are disproportionately
represented, a trend that reflects the historical presence of black, Asian,
and Latino men in certain realms of reproductive labor (Duffy 2007).

The men and women interviewed for this book possess demographic
characteristics that roughly mirror the general population of home care aides.
Of the thirty-three aides interviewed, twenty-eight are women and five are *sample data*
men. The sample is half white (sixteen respondents) and the remaining ra-
cial/ethnic breakdown is in line with the general population of aides in the
United States. Six of the interviewees are African American, four are Asian
American, five are Latino, and one person identifies as "mixed race." Ten of
the aides are foreign-born, and two are recently naturalized. To my knowledge, none of the workers are undocumented, although I did not discuss
immigration status extensively with participants. The diversity in the interview sample comes almost entirely from the California portion of the study.
In Ohio, all of aides interviewed were white women. This in part reflects the
demographic differences between the two states, but not entirely. Ohio has
a sizable population of African American direct care workers, but recruit-
ing these workers to participate in the study proved challenging. Method-
ological constraints notwithstanding, Ohio provides an important point of
contrast to California, as a state that has concentrated pockets of racial and
ethnic diversity in urban areas—largely composed of African Americans—
but is otherwise a very white, politically conservative, and economically
drained region (Lopez 2004). California stands in contrast to Ohio, as a state
with a sizable immigrant population and a rejuvenated labor movement
in some areas of the service sector (Mitchell 2004). As I discuss later, the core
components of aides' identity formation (i.e., the caring self) appear to tran-
scend geographic region. However, there are also observable differences in
the way in which aides of different racial and ethnic backgrounds conceive
of and narrate their care work, based largely on their own experiences with

discrimination. In this regard, there are important variations along lines of race and ethnicity that emerge when the California and Ohio workers are compared.

The elderly and disabled clients served by the aides in this study come from a range of racial, ethnic, and socioeconomic backgrounds. Some clients are middle class and "private pay," while others rely on state funding to pay for their care. In both California and Ohio, a number of the clients are Medicaid recipients, who are often poor and disproportionately likely to identify as a racial or ethnic minority. In the IHSS program in California, for example, 57 percent of the nearly three hundred thousand clients enrolled in 2002 identified as belonging to racial and ethnic minority groups (California Welfare Directors Association 2002). Workers interviewed in both states tend to care for clients of their own racial or ethnic backgrounds: only four of the aides interviewed were caring for a person of a race or ethnicity different from their own at the time of the interview. Over the course of a paid caring career, however, aides report working for clients outside their racial and ethnic group.

The bottom line is that the demographic profiles of both aides and their clients reflect broader inequalities tied to the organization of long-term care. As is the case with other forms of domestic labor, such as housecleaning or child care, more often than not poor women of color care for the elderly and disabled. Home care aides do differ from other domestic laborers in one important regard, however: they often care for people who—unlike middle- and upper-class men and women who hire a maid or a nanny—are disenfranchised by race, age, ability, or socioeconomic status. I assert that this makes the relationship between aide and client qualitatively different from that of maid and employer, or nanny and employer. When social hierarchy is blurred in an intimate dyad, as it is for aides and their clients, relationships are more apt to mimic informal caring bonds than formal ones. As a result, emotional connections—and the labor associated with those connections—become central to the story.

The Emotional Proletariat

When we consider factors like low wages, job insecurity, and the racialized nature of paid care work, it is clear that certain people—women, minorities—face structural disadvantages when caring in the service economy. In addition to these structural constraints, workers also face inequalities associated with the emotive, interactive demands of caring labor. Beginning with the work of Hochschild (1983), scholars have long considered the extent to which service work compels employees to evoke an emotional state in order to sell a product or provide a service (Ashforth and Humphrey 1993; Erickson and Wharton 1997; Gutek et al. 2000; Lopez 2006; Tolich 1993; Weaver 2005; Wharton 1993). This production of feeling, or emotional labor, can constrain or alienate the self, with potentially deleterious consequences for those who do the work of the "emotional proletariat" (Macdonald and Sirianni 1996).

To what extent paid caregivers, such as low-skilled health workers, experience alienation of self as a result of their emotional labor is an unanswered empirical question. Gaps in knowledge about emotion management among health care workers exist at both the top and bottom of the medical hierarchy; we know little about the way in which doctors on the one hand, and aides or "auxiliary" workers on the other, manage emotion at work (Erickson and Grove 2008). Rather, existing studies on emotional labor in health care focus largely on nurses, in part because they are the professional group most obviously responsible for the direct care of patients (Erickson and Grove 2008). While research on emotional labor in nursing constitutes an important contribution to the literature, the omission of low-skilled health care workers from the discussion of emotional labor is curious, especially considering that many other service workers have been considered, including telemarketers, waitresses, hairdressers, store clerks, and concierges (for exceptions to the omission of low-skilled health care workers, see Berdes and Eckert 2007 and Lopez 2006). What we do know from existing studies is that the *context* of work changes the meaning and experience of emotional labor for workers (Conradson 2003; Erickson and Grove 2008; Lopez 2006; Steinberg and Figart 1999). As such, it is necessary to consider how the emotion management of nursing aides conforms to or differs from the experiences of nurses, as well as other nonmedical workers in the service sector.

Even though the emotional labor of nursing aides has been largely understudied to date, those who research the long-term care workforce from an applied policy perspective indirectly address the subject in their investigations of burnout, depression, and stress among direct care workers.

We know, for example, that workers who face intense emotional demands in the workplace, especially nursing homes, are more likely to leave the job, become depressed, or experience burnout (Brannon et al. 2002; Muntaner 2006; Muntaner et al. 2006; R. Stone 2004). What remains unclear is the quality and context of these emotional demands and how these demands differ depending on whether an aide works in an institution or in a private home.

It is important to note that emotional labor is not always tied to poor outcomes for workers, including nursing aides. Lopez (2006) argues, for example, that organizational constraints—and the degree to which workers maneuver within these constraints—determine to a large extent whether emotional labor translates into positive or negative experiences for nursing aides working in institutional settings. Other studies of nursing aides support the more general assertion that affective ties to clients can be a source of job satisfaction, as well as a potential source of strain (Berdes and Eckert 2007; Chechin 1993; Neysmith and Aronson 1996). These findings are further corroborated by research in the broader literature on service workers that demonstrates the capacity of some employees to maneuver within, and glean meaning from, interpersonal pressures at work. Whether the subject of study is fast-food workers (Leidner 1991, 1999), mortuary science students (Cahill 1999), real estate agents (C. Wharton 1996), or service workers living in poverty (Newman 1999b), there is considerable evidence to suggest that some laborers extract meaning and positive self-concept from the interactive dimensions of work.

It is useful, when thinking through both the positive and negative implications of emotional labor, to think of emotions as *resources* (in the materialist sense of the word) as much as feelings or sentiments. The conceptualization of emotion as resource is central to Hochschild's (1983) original contribution. In her reading of emotional labor, affect is a resource extracted from workers by managers and owners who seek to sell a product or service, often at great detriment to an employee's sense of self. I contend that the vast research on emotional labor that has emerged subsequent to Hochschild's 1983 book has focused on the psychosocial outcomes and consequences of emotional labor at the expense of a materialist emphasis on emotions as resources. As some have noted, Hochschild included, the selective interpretation of emotional labor is in part tied to adoption of the concept by radically divergent disciplines and subfields, from social psychology with an emphasis on mental health outcomes, to business administration management where interest centers on emotional labor as a barrier to organizational efficacy (Hochschild 2003; Steinberg and Figart 1999).

The concept of "emotional capital," used largely by feminist scholars who analyze women's affective labor in the home, serves to remind us that emotions are indeed resources. Women's affective ties—to their children, their partners, their extended families—constitute a form of "emotional capital" that nurtures and sustains family bonds (Illouz 1997, 2007; Lovell 2000; Nowotny 1981; Reay 2004). Unlike other forms of capital—social, cultural—women's accrual of emotional capital does not usually result in greater access to economic capital or higher social status, precisely because it circulates within the confines of the family (Nowotny 1981; Reay 2004). So while women clearly amass emotional capital at rates greater than men—by providing care to children and elders, by maintaining ties to friends and neighbors, by investing time in their child's school and extracurricular activities—the resource does not hold much currency or social value beyond the private sphere, or so the literature suggests (Nowotny 1981). The concept of emotional capital, then, dovetails nicely with Hochschild's discussion of emotional labor, since in either case emotions are presented as resources that can be extracted from women to produce inequality in both public (workplace) and private (family) spheres.

Social psychologists offer a slightly different interpretation of emotional capital, one that considers the role emotions play in both social interaction and the construction of identity. Cahill (1999) identifies emotional capital as a set of biographical characteristics that predispose individuals—in his particular study, mortuary science students—to deftly handle emotionally charged or demanding situations. He argues that emotional socialization in childhood and later life (i.e., secondary socialization) leads to the accumulation of emotional capital, which partly explains why certain people end up in jobs that require emotion management and why these same people often view themselves as gifted in or destined to do such work. Cahill makes clear that emotional capital is not solely a function of individual biography, arguing instead that capital accumulates in relation to one's social location, such as one's race, class, and gender (113). Women, for example, are socialized to be caregivers from an early age, building significant emotional capital along the way. While this emotional socialization certainly produces a gendered division of labor in both the home and workplace (Chodorow 1978), Cahill reminds us that emotions are also important resources that enable workers to deftly manage human interaction while on the job.

Returning to the empirical example of nursing aides, it is clear from the interviews with workers in Ohio and California that women, and a few men, accumulate a great deal of emotional capital before entering paid caregiving. Aides in this study, with no exceptions, have years of informal caring experience—caring for sick spouses or parents, providing for the needs of their children (and sometimes their grandchildren), or tending to the needs of friends and neighbors. Describing themselves in terms such as "the only one who cares," "the caregiver in the family," "the person people turn to," or "a natural caregiver," aides allude to the fact that years of providing for family prepared them for a career in paid care work. Once on the job, aides report utilizing their emotional capital to navigate—and draw meaning from—their interpersonal relationships with clients. While aides view their emotional capital in overwhelmingly positive terms—as the very thing that makes them good at what they do—it is important to remember that this capital carries little advantage in terms of monetary compensation or social validation. As such, emotions in the context of low-skilled care work can be viewed simultaneously as resources that aides utilize to construct identity on the job, as well as resources that agencies extract from workers in exchange for a meager wage and, often, poor working conditions. Put more succinctly, emotions in the context of paid care work produce *identity* while also reinforcing *inequality*.

Caring Trajectories and Emotional Capital

Emotional capital accrues in the lives of home care aides, and arguably other low-skilled caregivers, as they move between informal (unpaid) and formal (paid) care work. Interviews with aides in California and Ohio provide evidence of a clear caring trajectory that begins with the informal care of family or friends and leads, at some point, to a job in direct care. The caring trajectories of the thirty-three aides interviewed for this book are strikingly similar, even though the sample varies considerably by race, ethnicity, and geographic location of work. Below I introduce two aides:

Tiffany, a forty-eight-year-old white woman who works for Maximum Care in Ohio, and Jackie, a forty-two-year-old African American woman who works in California. Although it is difficult to imagine that these women have much in common—at least in terms of personal history and geographic location—their caring trajectories run parallel in a number of ways. Both women have a history of caring for family and see themselves as "natural" caregivers, both have moved in and out of paid care work, and both see themselves as having strong emotional skills (emotional capital) that allow them to do the job well. Predictably, they also struggle in similar ways to make ends meet.

Tiffany

Tiffany has lived and worked in the same town in northern Ohio for most of her life. During high school, in the 1970s, Tiffany worked in a nursing home, preparing and serving food to elderly residents. Within a few years of graduation, Tiffany got married and had two children. Divorced only a few years later, Tiffany found herself in need of work and decided to provide child care in her own home so that she could care for her own kids during the day. Once her children were school-age, Tiffany decided to return to the nursing home where she had worked as a teen to receive on-the-job training as a licensed state tested nursing assistant (STNA). After she became certified, Tiffany remained in nursing home care, earning minimum wage for over twenty years, taking breaks from the job for short stints (six months to a year). As Tiffany explained to me, even though conditions at nursing homes frustrate her (it is not uncommon for Tiffany to be in charge of twenty patients per shift) she "always goes back."

When she is asked about her reasons for working in facilities, it is clear that Tiffany has limited options when it comes to gainful employment and that nursing homes bring with them a certain security in the form of predictable work hours and, usually, health benefits. She has worked in a rubber factory, a metal factory, and a plastic factory, as well as holding other service jobs (flower arranger in a grocery store and McDonald's server, for example). While these service jobs were relatively free of emotional strain, particularly compared to nursing work, Tiffany found herself seeking out opportunities to "connect" with customers in ways that just were not possible in the context. For example, while working at McDonald's, Tiffany enjoyed serving senior citizens, sometimes helping them to their tables and pausing for a minute to chat. Speaking of her various jobs in the service industry, Tiffany remarks, "I liked the thought that you still get to talk to people and stuff, but it wasn't the same…you just can't do that [develop relationships]." On her most recent hiatus from the nursing home, Tiffany decided to look for work in home care. She now juggles shifts between home care and a nursing facility for Alzheimer's patients, but has a strong preference for home care, which she finds more "personal" and "one-on-one."

Tiffany's caring trajectory, like that of so many women I interviewed, began in her youth. Tiffany shared in the care of a "troubled" brother throughout her teenage years. After navigating life as a single mom and family child care provider in her twenties, Tiffany became responsible for managing her mother's long deterioration from Alzheimer's. Soon after her mother passed away, Tiffany cared for her father as he died of colon cancer. Although Tiffany's two children are out of the home, she now helps her sister who is disabled and cannot drive, while also running errands and caring for her nephew who is bipolar and low functioning. Like many of the women I interviewed, Tiffany juggles the demands of informal caregiving while also dealing with the emotional and physical stresses of her paid care work. Tiffany reports there are days when balancing family and work prove difficult but that she simply perseveres: "Sometimes it gets to me. But I think I still have more days where I just do it, because it is something I've always done. It's like a natural thing for me.…I guess some say I'm just a person who's like a caretaker; I just take care of everything."

Tiffany acknowledges the stress that comes from being the family caregiver, but she also recognizes that she has accrued an impressive emotional skill set in twenty-five years of taking care of others. Tiffany talked to me about her ability to comfort grieving people, her techniques for eliciting a response from patients with dementia, and her knack for calming down agitated or distressed clients. She spoke of one occasion in particular, while moonlighting in a group home for mentally retarded adults, when one of the residents became very agitated and physically aggressive, to such a degree that other staff could not restrain her. Tiffany was clocking on to her shift as the situation escalated and describes walking into the room, sitting down next to the resident in question and looking her straight in the eye and greeting her in a calm, reassuring voice. Within minutes, Tiffany recalls, the resident composed herself and expressed delight that Tiffany had arrived. When I prompted Tiffany to articulate exactly what she did right in the situation, she responded: "You just have to know how to treat people. You just can't treat people like little kids, and you can't argue with them. You just have to know how to *be* with them."

Jackie

Jackie has worked as a CNA in Central City, California, for nearly ten years. Like Tiffany, Jackie's experiences caring for family and friends extend well into her youth. As we talked on the sofa in her home, Jackie explained how she developed a reputation as an informal caregiver, largely as a result of the many years she spent providing support to family and friends in the neighborhood. Jackie is very active in her church, which is where she formed a relationship with her first client, Bettie, an elderly woman who had moved to Central City from Baltimore, but learned soon after that she had cancer. With no family nearby or friends to speak of, and anticipating her need for help, Bettie asked Jackie if she would check on her daily during chemotherapy and radiation treatments. "Checking in" turned into nearly full-time caregiving, as Jackie became Bettie's support system in her last months and weeks of life. Jackie received no monetary compensation for Bettie's care, but did realize that she had a talent for caring, and that she was not "put off" by bodily fluids and the emotional stress of caring for an ill person as some of her sisters were. After Bettie died, Jackie continued to provide care, occasionally for pay, to other elderly members of her church. Although she found the work fulfilling, Jackie needed to contribute more money to the family budget, so she found a job at a nursing home and received on-the-job training to become a CNA. Since then, Jackie has worked largely in home-based care, believing that the pace and demands of institutions precludes "personal time" with patients, something she feels is very important.

Jackie currently lives with three of her sisters, her mother, her daughter, and her young grandson, and has done so for as long as she can remember. Men have been in and out of Jackie's life, including her own father, and she describes her immediate and extended family as "mostly women." Having so many family members under one roof has proved particularly important in the last year, since Jackie's mother was diagnosed with incurable lung cancer. Jackie and her siblings organize their work schedules so that someone is always at home with their mother, who is on oxygen and generally very weak. Jackie is proud of her family's commitment to caring for kin, describing in detail the ways that they rally around their mother when her spirits are low or her treatments are particularly grueling. The family has even taken to sleeping together on the living room floor some nights, with her mother on the couch, so they can all comfort her when she awakes in the night, disoriented from her medications. Jackie believes that she has "trained" her eight-year-old grandson to care for others. He has responded by taking an active interest in the well-being of his grandmother, often administering medicine or changing her oxygen. We talked about the possibility that he might also find a career in paid caregiving, although Jackie seems amused at the prospect of a young man doing the work she does.

Jackie believes she will be in home care for the rest of her working life, even though the low pay means that Jackie's contribution to the family purse is relatively small. To compensate, the family continues to pool its resources, which enables Jackie to stay in a job that she identifies as a "calling" and a "gift from God." Since home care is also more flexible in terms of when hours are worked, Jackie's choice of employment ensures that she can take the lead in organizing her mother's care.

When I ask Jackie to elaborate about her "gift" for caregiving, she says she possesses an ability to connect emotionally with sick or elderly people otherwise ignored by family members or medical personnel who don't have the time to give. She tells me:

> I think when you are sick like that, you need special attention, and you need that hands-on....They just need someone there just to talk, and that helps them, and they heal. To me it's the inside healing that you need first, and that's what I look at.

Jackie believes her emotional investment in patients also benefits her in the long term: "I think God is going to reward me greatly. That is it, and that's why I'm in it, because it is a gift from him and I know he's going to reward me."

The caring trajectories of Jackie and Tiffany are strikingly similar, even though the specifics of their life circumstances vary considerably. Both women provide a significant amount of informal care to their families, and have done so from an early age. The two women also describe their transitions from unpaid to paid care work in similar ways, as obvious and seamless extensions of the work they do for their families. Finally, both view themselves as possessing a God-given or natural ability to care. While they have cycled in and out of aide jobs, often in search of better pay, both Tiffany and Jackie view their paid care work as a "calling" that is difficult to walk away from.

Tiffany and Jackie, like most people, view their caring histories through the lens of personal, rather than group, experience. When considered on the aggregate, however, the caring trajectories of almost all of the aides I spent time with display the same basic pattern: paid care work follows from, and often coincides with, extensive care work demands in the family. Sociologists of gender would find such a statement unsurprising, as they have long studied the gendered division of labor in the home and how this form of inequality penalizes women in the labor force, in the form of wage gaps, occupational segregation, and the much-discussed glass ceiling (Jacobs and Gerson 2004). Scholars of care work have refined this analysis further, asserting that informal caregivers, especially those who are older and low skilled, are more likely to suffer job loss and wage gaps as a result of caring demands at home (Wakabayashi and Donato 2005, 2006). For those women who then enter paid caring careers, the projections for wages and mobility are even bleaker since there is a clear wage penalty associated with paid care work (England, Budig, and Folbre 2002).

It is clear that the structural realities of women's work, both paid and unpaid, translate into clear disadvantages for paid care workers, especially in terms of wages and job mobility. This structural inequality arguably manifests on a microinteractional level, as heavy affective demands exact a psychosocial toll on aides, with little material reward. Throughout this book, one will find ample evidence to support the broad assertion that low-waged care work exacerbates existing inequalities of race, class, and gender, fostering a racial and gendered division of labor.

Given the link between care work and inequality, what do we make of Tiffany and Jackie, who view their emotional commitments to clients in an overwhelmingly positive light? How do we interpret the empirical finding that, for these and other caregivers, emotional exploitation does not obviously follow from material exploitation? To make sense of aides' subjective experience of caregiving, it is useful to consider how identity forms in the *context* of inequality. Doing so helps theorize the myriad ways in which social actors maneuver within the structural constraints of a service economy (low wages, lack of mobility, decreased autonomy). To link identity and inequality in this way also calls on, and contributes to, emerging scholarship in the area of care work that considers how women narrate and make decisions about their paid and unpaid caring commitments in the face of limited choices (Macdonald 2010; P. Stone 2007; Tuominen 2003).

Returning to Tiffany and Jackie, both characterize their ability to relate to elderly clients as innate and natural, part of an "authentic" sense of self (Erickson 1995). Although the women tend to narrate their care as natural, these perceptions belie a broader history of familial and gendered obligations to care, limited job prospects, and poor job mobility. At the same time, these aides possess an emotional skill set, or emotional capital, that affords them a certain degree of expertise and competency on the job. Tiffany's gift for "being with people" and Jackie's commitment to the "inside healing" of her patients further suggest that the skills associated with being an aide are largely emotional and relational rather than physical or technical. It is not surprising, then, that aides' presentation of self—what I call the caring self—is so closely tied to their emotional experiences and emotion management in client homes. The point here is that while structural inequality clearly limits workers' life chances, the women themselves call on very traditional, gendered understandings of caregiving to establish their social value and preserve a sense of self on the job. This "identity work" plays a role in restoring dignity to a job often viewed as low skilled or dirty. This is not to say that aides do not experience some very real constraints while caring for clients. As the following chapters illustrate, there is considerable physical and emotional labor associated with home care.

2

Doing the Dirty Work

The Physical and Emotional Labor of Home Care

VIRGINIA

For the last thirty years, Virginia has been taking care of other people for a wage. A white woman in her early sixties, Virginia is tall and appears very muscular, characteristics that are somewhat at odds with her gentle manner and tone of voice. Her work history includes the care of elderly adults with chronic illness (both in and out of nursing homes), children with autism, developmentally disabled adults, and middle-class children in need of a nanny. Some of her clients have been wealthy, or "gold coast," as she puts it, but the vast majority have been poor and elderly. Over time, Virginia has accrued very little economic capital—she still struggles to pay the bills at the end of each month and has no retirement to speak of other than Social Security—but prides herself on her ability to walk into a home "cold" and develop trusting relationships with complete strangers. This emotional capital has served Virginia well over the years, getting her out of "sticky" emotional situations with clients, such as the time she reported her elderly client to the agency because he was regularly taking five pills for his heart condition rather than the prescribed two, at great risk to his health. Feeling she had violated the terms of their bond, the elderly client subjected Virginia to three weeks of the silent treatment before she could coax him to trust her again. Such stories (and characters) are a common part of Virginia's work life and part of the reason she likes the job.

Now sixty-two, Virginia continues to work as an aide and plans to do so well into retirement. Her ability to connect with clients notwithstanding, Virginia finds the work both emotionally and physically draining. Ten years ago, Virginia had surgery on her colon and went back to work early in her recovery, in need of income. Lifting a client, she triggered a series of injuries to her surgery site, as well as to her back. Unemployed for a brief period after her injury, Virginia eventually found work managing properties for a local company. Although the work paid fairly well, certainly better than home care, Virginia eventually returned to her job as an aide. As she puts it, "Oh yeah, being in home care...you know, it's funny...I guess I've just learned to love it because it's a different [job], it's just different. I'm trying to leave it and I just never can seem to leave it. I'm still here."

Like Virginia, many of the aides talk about the work of home care as being "different" from other service jobs, to the point that they find themselves continually cycling back into home-based work after periods of unemployment or after stints in other lines of work. Despite its allure, it is also clear that there are physical and emotional demands associated with this type of caregiving, some of which exact a considerable toll on workers.

Home Care versus Institutional Care

To date, aides working in facilities have received considerable attention from sociologists, gerontologists, and scholars of long-term care (Berdes and Eckert 2007; Diamond 1992; Foner 1994; Lopez 2006). In contrast, research on home-based aides is relatively scant, and what exists tends to be quantitative and largely descriptive (Crown, Ahlburg, and MacAdam 1995; Paraprofessional Healthcare Institute 2008c; Yamada 2002). This omission is partially a function of history. In the 1990s, at the height of the crisis over mismanagement and elder abuse in nursing facilities, scholars and policymakers directed attention to the poor working conditions and declining quality of care in long-term care facilities (Foner 1994; Institute of Medicine of the National Academies 2008). In the context of this policy crisis, sociologists responded with ethnographic investigations of nursing homes in an effort to understand how bureaucratic norms and for-profit logic fuels both worker disaffection and the mistreatment of clients in institutional settings (Diamond 1992; Foner 1994).

Ethnographic work changed the discussion about long-term care in two important ways. First, ethnographers like Foner (1994) and Diamond (1992) tell the story of nursing homes by shifting focus from the perspective of patients to the perspective of aides caring for them. Prior to this, rich accounts of aides' experiences were largely absent from both scholarly and policy research on nursing homes. Second, the work of Foner and Diamond directs attention to the benefits of studying paid caregiving in situ, qualitatively and ethnographically, so that aides' commitments and orientations to their work are fully understood within the context of their lives, work environments, and relationships to others. Home care aides arguably require a similar qualitative treatment of their experiences, so that scholars of long-term care can begin to recognize the full scope of work that aides do, and how this differs from work done by their counterparts in nursing homes.

Perhaps few researchers consider whether or how home care aides differ from other long-term care workers because, on the surface, the occupational locations and work tasks of aides in home and institutional settings appear identical. Both sites of care attract large numbers of women, offer little in the way of job advancement or training, provide few health benefits, and take a great physical and emotional toll (Hollander Feldman 1994). However, interviews and observations of home care aides reveal some important distinctions between home-based and institutional aides. This difference centers on the greater ratio of emotional to physical labor expected of home care workers, and the blurring of boundaries between work and family, ever present in home care. In the pages that follow,

I present worker descriptions of home care, detailing how paid caregiving taxes aides financially, physically, and emotionally.

Conditions of Work: Financial and Physical Strains

Aides providing home care generally earn less than their counterparts working in nursing homes or other institutions. In addition, home care aides often work without health or retirement benefits, are subjected to unpredictable work hours, and can suffer injury providing hands-on care. Although aides in this study generally opt for home-based work, actively avoiding institutional care, they nonetheless feel constrained by the many stresses and strains of the job.

Maggie, a sixty-two-year-old white aide, was recently forced to retire after thirty years of providing home care to hundreds of elderly clients in northeast Ohio. Only months before we met, Maggie had been in a serious car accident that left her with a chronic and painful back injury. Unable to lift or move around without experiencing pain, Maggie quit her job as a home care aide and, without the means to pay rent, gave up the apartment she had been living in for ten years. Soon after, she moved into a retirement home for low-income seniors, the only place she could afford with her meager Social Security income. Maggie talked at length about how quickly the tables had turned for her—from being a caregiver to someone in need of care—and said that she has very few people or financial resources to draw on for help. Without health insurance, for example, Maggie must rely for now on community clinics to treat her back injury, while she waits out the next few years until she is eligible for Medicare. When I ask Maggie to reflect on her current vulnerability, given the years she has spent caring for others, she comments, "I mean, it's not right. It isn't. You dedicate your whole life to taking care of people, then there's nothing for you. You just put so much in, and you get very little back."

For other aides, it is the unpredictable nature of the work, as well as the need to juggle multiple clients to make ends meet, that results in considerable work stress. Some clock forty-, fifty-, even sixty-hour workweeks in order to make a living. Virginia, mentioned above, is thankful that she has seen her wages go from four dollars an hour in the late 1970s to $9.50 today, but emphasizes that when travel time and gas money are factored in (none of which are compensated), her real wage is insufficient, especially given the number of clients she juggles in a day, four on average. Beyond inadequate pay, Virginia finds the unpredictable nature of home-based care taxing, both physically and emotionally. Since clients sometimes end up in the hospital (or, in better circumstances, go away on vacation), aides like Virginia can, without notice, find themselves with lighter workloads and less income for weeks at a time:

> I was down hours and sometimes I'd get calls, sometimes I wouldn't. And I just couldn't face my bills and things. It was hard on me. My stomach would be torn up. And in a forty-hour week you could be canceled and they end up going in the hospital. Some of them decide to take vacation, you know, many things can happen, and if they [the agency] don't have anyone to fill in, your living is going up and down and it's very insecure.

Most aides accept with little complaint the financial constraints of the job, emphasizing instead the symbolic value of caregiving, a topic I discuss at length in chapter 3. Interestingly, aides tend not to blame the agencies in a global sense for low wages, viewing the business's profit motive as legitimate and necessarily at odds with higher wages for workers. Aides do, however, find fault with decisions made by management at individual agencies. Shelly, a twenty-eight-year-old white aide, described situations where she was asked by her employer (an agency) to tend to a client on her day off, never receiving compensation for the work because she was ineligible for overtime. Kristen, a sixty-five-year-old white aide, complained that her employer pays her wages via a prepaid Visa card, one that comes with a monthly maintenance fee that she is responsible for and that charges her each time she attempts to access cash from the account. Even though Kristen requested a check for her wages rather than the Visa card, the employer claimed this was impossible. Kristen estimated that she loses twenty dollars a month (two hours of wages) as a result of the agency's payroll system.

On-the-job injuries are fairly commonplace among aides, if the experiences of the men and women in this study are a good indication of larger workforce trends. Although the injuries tend to be chronic rather than acute, and rarely lead to sustained unemployment, aides in the study do identify physical strain and injury as a persistent stressor. Back strain, of the variety that forced Maggie into retirement, was the most commonly cited injury, usually the result of improperly "transferring" a client from one place or position in the house to another (a bed to a chair, for example). For some, such an injury is temporarily debilitating; for others it is an ongoing nuisance with which they simply cope.

Joyce, an African American aide in her early seventies, is now caring for her ailing brother, who is dying of cancer. Joyce is paid by IHSS to tend to her brother, but has worked as a home care aide for nonrelatives. After her brother "passes," Joyce tells me she will likely find another client to care for, since she has little in the way of retirement funds. Joyce continues to work as an aide, despite a chronic back injury she sustained ten years prior while caring for an elderly woman in Texas for six dollars an hour. She described to me the circumstances of the injury and the problems she had finding adequate medical care:

> So this particular morning, I take her to the potty. I was sitting her on the potty-chair, and then instead of her going to the potty-chair, she went the other way, which means that I had to go the other way and pull some muscles in my body. As an end result of that, I didn't work anymore [with this client]. In February I went to a doctor, a chiropractor, and of course the insurance bucked, I mean really bucked. The doctors did not act in my behalf, saying that I could go back to work, and I couldn't go back to work. So then...I went to physical therapy and...when I found out how much it was costing! It cost three hundred some dollars for me to go there for an hour, and I'm saying, Wait a minute, he's not doing that much good. I stopped going to physical therapy and I still have problems with my back.

Public health research on the home care workforce suggests that injuries like Joyce's are not uncommon and that injured aides tend to "work through it" or cycle through periods of unemployment as a way of managing the injury, rather than filing for workers' compensation or some other form of financial support (Scherzer and Wolfe 2008). Aides who work informally for clients, rather than contracting with an agency, find themselves in a particularly precarious position once injured. These workers, as a rule, have no health benefits and are ineligible for workers' compensation.

The Space of Work

Since home care takes place in private space, it is not surprising that some of the stress, as well as the rewards, stem from the variable physical conditions in which aides work. While the majority of aides enjoy the informal and familiar environs of a home, there are times when home-based work proves stressful, even hazardous. Maggie, mentioned earlier in this chapter, worked for an elderly woman with Alzheimer's who needed around-the-clock care. The woman's home was filled with animal feces from cats and dogs still in the home. Caring for an elderly woman was the least demanding aspect of her job, Maggie said, as she described the unsanitary and even threatening environment in which she worked:

> I had a client over in Middletown. The lady had Alzheimer's, which I dealt with. It was no problem. People were filthy, nasty, they had animals all in their house, feces. The son, which was lazy, he was a bum. Lived off of his parents. Cats, dogs, all through the house. Urine all through the home. Feces everywhere from the animals. Just filth. And the guy that lived there, the son, had a gun laid on the table. I put up with that for a year. I felt like I was being threatened. All the time he would bring it out. And they told us we didn't have to put up with them. Well, I complained and complained and complained, I finally got away from that environment. Because I felt I was being threatened, and I told her son, "I'm not here for you; I'm here for the care of your mother. I'm not a crook. I'm not a housekeeper. These are my duties. I'm not supposed to wait on you." I put up with that for a year. I was scared to death. I never experienced nothing like that. I said, "Don't ever ask me to come back, because I'm not." He was a nasty person. Oh, it was awful. I felt so uncomfortable. I just, I said, "I'll never go back there. Never."

For other aides, it is not the physical conditions or work environment that pose a problem, but the fact that they live near their clients, often in the same neighborhood or on the same block. This close proximity to one's "workplace" has obvious benefits (workers do not have to commute or spend wages on transportation), but it can also produce both physical and emotional strain. Tammy, a fifty-one-year-old white aide living near Middletown, Ohio, spent the first three or four years of her home care career working for a woman who lived next door to her. Tammy and her client, Sue, were mere acquaintances until Sue's multiple sclerosis moved into an acute phase. Living alone, Sue asked her neighbors whether they knew of anyone who could provide daily care for a wage. Tammy, a stay-at-home wife and mother, offered her services and, over a four-year period, became

Sue's primary caregiver. Tammy described her physical proximity to Sue in this way:

> We lived right next door. And it was physically, geographically, logistically hard to separate. You know, I would listen during the summer when the windows were open. We could hear Sue. I mean, she could actually yell out the window if she needed me.

Tammy is passionate about her work as a home care aide and believes, as many of the aides do, that the work is a "calling," something she was born to do. Even so, Tammy found it frustrating at times to live so close to the woman for whom she cared, since it made it nearly impossible for her to establish clear boundaries between work and home. As she put it, "I guess now that I think of it...I think I was pretty much on call 24/7 for all those years."

Too Much Responsibility, Too Little Training

Broader changes to the organization of health care in the United States have a direct impact on low-skilled workers such as home care aides. Increased pressure to meet the demand side of long-term care (i.e., the growing number of elderly and disabled who seek in-home care) means that private and public agencies struggle to find enough workers to send into the field. As a result, training is often an afterthought. As one aide commented, "You just need a pulse" in order to get a job as a home care aide.

By all accounts, the work of being an aide, at least in a home setting, generally requires very little formal medical training. Agencies, if they provide any training at all, will ask aides to attend a brief workshop where they might watch a video about universal precautions and learn when and how to call for medical assistance in the case of an emergency. In one instance, for example, an aide described watching an obviously dated video in a closet-size room of an agency with five other aides and no facilitator. Some agencies send home care aides in their employ yearly "exams" in the mail to test basic safety skills. Aides describe these as easy to fill out, not very challenging, and unrelated to the day-to-day challenges they face on the job. Aides working for IHSS in Central City, California, are unionized members of SEIU (Service Employees International Union), giving them access to better training, such as workshops on nutrition, transferring (lifting) clients, or managing the stress of caregiving.[1] In general, though, aides complain that trainings are infrequent and cursory, leaving them feeling relatively unprepared for the emotional demands of the work or a possible medical emergency.

It almost goes without saying that when you work with an elderly or chronically ill person, medical emergencies are bound to arise. As a result, most aides find themselves in situations beyond their training at one time or another. Aides describe these moments as intensely frightening, primarily because they feel trapped between wanting to act (giving someone CPR, for example) and knowing that agencies severely restrict aides from performing any medical hands-on care of clients, even in the case of an emergency. Tammy, from Middletown, Ohio, describes the problem in this way:

> The agency can send an aide with only basic office training or agency training....[The training] doesn't even involve taking blood pressure. I mean, the health training is very minimal. But they could...send me to a very involved patient with hands-on medical needs, who needs help with medications, which we're not trained to do. And you get in some really dangerous situations there for the aide and the client, physically and legally. So I'm very uneasy about it....I don't feel I'm trained to take those difficult patients. If they can't find anyone else, I do. But I don't like it.

In fact, Tammy found herself in two precarious situations in the last few years, where she felt compelled to provide medical care beyond the scope of her training. In the first instance, Tammy was caring for a very frail elderly man who was paralyzed, unable to stand or walk, but who needed to be lifted regularly from bed to be washed. The agency alerted Tammy to the client's condition and asked her to watch a short video that included a five-minute segment on transferring patients. Tammy nervously agreed to take the case after seeing the video, but when faced with the reality of moving a paralyzed man whose body was taller and heavier than hers, she realized the limits of her training. Frightened, Tammy "somehow" moved the client from his bed into the shower, only to realize that he could not balance himself and that putting any pressure on his fragile skin was causing him to bruise and feel pain. Tammy remembers the incident in detail:

T: He had, you know, his skin was extremely fragile. I'd bathed people, but you can't just bathe that kind of person; there's a specific

CS: procedure. And he needed special soaps and special cloths. Some of
those are just frightening.

CS: Did you say, "I can't do this"?

T: I didn't. His wife was there. If she hadn't been there to tell me
what to do, I wouldn't have done it. I did say, "You have to stay
with me. You have to tell me exactly what to do. I'm afraid I'll hurt
him." And she did, and it went fine. But it was really stressful. And
the poor guy, he doesn't know me from, you know, Eve. And he
was very understanding. But I could tell that I hurt him. And that's
just unacceptable.

On a second occasion, Tammy was caring for her neighbor, Sue, when
the visiting nurse failed to show up for a regular visit. Sue's catheter had
become very uncomfortable and badly needed "flushing," something that
Tammy had seen done on a training video years earlier but that she understood as an "off-limits" procedure because of her limited training. Sue
pleaded with Tammy to remove and drain the catheter. Tammy agonized
over the decision for an hour, weighing the potential consequences of her
actions in her head. Finally, after several calls to the visiting nurse went
unreturned, Tammy decided to remove the catheter and flush it. Reinsert-
ing it proved difficult, however, and after several failed attempts Tammy
called the paramedics. Frightened and a bit embarrassed by the incident,
Tammy talked about feeling torn between acting quickly to meet her client's urgent needs and feeling constrained by a vague set of rules that prohibit her from performing most medical tasks. Although Tammy worked
on a private basis for Sue—and was therefore not beholden to a set of formal rules and procedures set forth by an agency—she nonetheless believed
she would be held liable if something were to go wrong. Tammy feels her
lack of training, along with her fear of negative repercussions, prevents
her from acting in the larger interests of her clients:

> If I know how to do it, and I'm confident, I think I'm very good at caregiv-
> ing. But if I'm not confident—being nervous and having the shaking hand
> can make a huge difference on somebody's body. No, I would just love it
> [training]. For example, I'm CPR certified. And yet I have never heard of an
> agency that requires that. And I'm not certain that if I did perform CPR on
> a client, I may be immediately dismissed. I mean, that may be grounds for
> termination. Even a lawsuit. Especially if it wasn't successful.

Jennifer, a white aide in her midfifties working in California, was given a great deal of latitude to monitor and treat her client's diabetes, even though she was not completely comfortable with this arrangement. She recounts a story of the time that the client's public health nurse "ordered" Jennifer to manage insulin injections:

> So I talked to the nurse and she said, "Well, do this, this, and this, and if this happens, then do this and this," and so it's just a matter of following the directions that were given to me. And she says, "Well, have you been doing this?" I said, "Hey, you know, it's not up to me to make that kind of a decision." I said, "I'm a home care provider, and I'm not medically trained, I'm not an RN, and it's not my discretion to do these things," and she said, "Well, we're giving it your discretion." I went, "Okay."

Jennifer displays some hesitation to take on work she is not trained to do, and her caution is not unwarranted; if something were to happen to her client, Jennifer would be held liable. Unlike physicians and nurses, Jennifer does her work without organizational protection and oversight. Seeing herself as the only person available to meet her client's needs, Jennifer is willing to take on this risk largely because she feels a deep connection to her client, an elderly woman in her eighties.

Andrew, a fifty-three-year-old African American man who has worked in home care in California for over ten years, explains that helping clients with their medical needs comes naturally to him after years of watching and learning on the job. He suggests that the agencies are fully aware of the fact that aides often do work that they are not formally trained to do:

> It's not in agreement with the agency, but they know we do a lot of things personally for our clients, because once you're with a client for four or five years, you know, you establish a kind of rapport with them, a friendship and trust, all this stuff is there. I had one, Ken, he's a very wealthy man, and I did just about everything for him.

Mark, an Asian American caregiver in his midforties working in Central City, confirms that in the IHSS program, aides often do more hands-on medical care than public health nurses, even though PHNs are some of the most highly trained registered nurses in the field. Mark, unlike Tammy and other caregivers discussed above, seems relatively unconcerned that he takes on medical work beyond his training and jurisdiction.

> In-home support [aides] can get away with more things because they do not have the censorship or the people that they have to report to all the time. Literally and legally, if you had four and five different medications that you had to take, I could literally lay them out and so forth, and have you take them. And maybe even illegally, but legally place them in your mouth because you needed help. Whereas an RN is not qualified to do it. Even though I'm not [an RN], I could get away with it and I'd have more range and variance, whereas an RN, they have to be put under constant microscope, having to report to everything and everybody. And so basically we can do almost the same things they can to a certain degree, we just don't need—we can get away with it without the training.

Aides who have been in the field for over twenty years remark that the situation with respect to training has changed considerably over the years. Dot, a fifty-one-year-old white aide, has been working in home care since her early thirties. Early in her career as an aide, she worked for a small, locally owned firm in Middletown, Ohio, run by two women who had turned from nursing to start their own home care business. Dot recalls strong camaraderie among workers and management, reinforced by continuing-education seminars and monthly employee meetings where aides would discuss problems they were facing on the job. For Dot, these meetings were invaluable, providing her with an opportunity to network with other aides and to learn more about the company for which she worked, Harmony Care. Not surprisingly, Dot made little money working for the company (her wage was just over four dollars per hour in the late 1980s), but she stuck it out because, in her own words, the owner made her feel as if she was "part of the company."

Dot compared her co-workers at Harmony Care to family, which explains why she says she "probably stayed longer, even with all the aggravation, the pay, and everything else." Since leaving Harmony Care fifteen years ago, Dot has worked for a series of large for-profit home care companies, including Maximum Care, and expresses frustration that the "mom-and-pop" feel of agencies no longer exists. Dot's anecdotal observation is supported by data on the home care industry, which suggests that in the last twenty years, the United States has seen unprecedented growth in for-profit home care (Institute of Medicine of the National Academies 2008;

Kaye et al. 2006). Despite this growth, few resources go to on-the-job train-ing, if the accounts offered by aides in Middletown and Central City are any indication. As a result, aides find themselves in situations where they must administer medication or change a catheter, sometimes without the proper training or equipment to do so.

The real question is, why are aides like Jennifer and Andrew assuming such risk? As a result of the changing medical landscape, where for-profit health care and the de-skilling of health work affect the nature and quality of care received, Jennifer and others like her assume the burden (and risk) of care because they are structurally positioned to do so. At the bottom of the medical hierarchy, aides are part of a frontline workforce, left to care for chronically ill elderly and disabled Americans. Aides come into close contact with clients who require skilled care but who often lack the economic resources or social ties (i.e., family) to secure it. In these circumstances, aides become nurses by default, taking on tasks outside of their training and jurisdiction.

Working within Bureaucratic Constraints

Although some aides, like Tammy above, worry that their limited training places them in precarious situations with respect to hands-on care, other aides express frustration that they are constrained by bureaucratic rules that prevent them from utilizing the skills they do have. In particular, aides working in the field for more than fifteen years lament the onslaught of bureaucratic rules and regulations that preclude them from fully caring for their patients. Many of these more experienced aides secured training in a different era of homecare, when hands-on care of clients, including wound care, CPR, and administration of medicine, was permitted, encouraged, and supported by agencies that tended to provide workers with training on minor medical procedures.

Dot, for example, remembers a time when she could administer medi-cation intravenously, after receiving training to do the task. Now, she re-ports, "I'm not allowed to give an aspirin." Dawn, a thirty-eight-year-old white aide, finds herself in a similar situation, although she has mixed feel-ings about whether bureaucratic restrictions on care, and the resultant de-skilling of her work, are ultimately a good or bad thing:

> In a way, it's nice because you don't have all this headache, you don't have all this gear to carry. I used to carry a bag that was sixteen times the size of

yours. I'm not kidding. We carried our wheelies [medical carts] and had everything in it. You name it, we carried it. And to go from that to a little clip-
board and gloves in my pocket, it's kind of nice—then you don't have all this
mess to contain. But, at the same time, nobody cares if you know how to do
that [medical work], and if you get caught doing it, you are out of a job.

Even younger home care aides, many of whom received CNA certification
in nursing homes, feel constrained by rules laid out by home care agencies.
Shelly, an aide in her midtwenties, says that restrictions on what aides cannot do "is one of the things that stinks about my job…because I have all
this training and it doesn't matter. I'm not even allowed to do CPR."

Of course, there is another side to the story about bureaucratic constraints facing workers. Precisely because home care agencies require very
little training, they must protect client safety by limiting the medical care
provided by aides. Liability issues are always looming for agency owners,
who must hire relatively unskilled workers to keep costs low and preserve
profit. Restricting aides' scope of work is the way in which agencies formally protect themselves from issues of liability that they will inevitably
face when minimally supervised caregivers provide services in the context
of a home. One home-care-agency owner describes problems of liability
that arise:

> Sometimes you have somebody doing an eight-hour day shift for you that's
> coming off a night shift and hasn't slept, and so their work is substandard or
> they fall asleep on the job, and the family complains. So you have all those
> problems that come out that need to be fixed.… Then we found out that an-
> other big barrier is that many times they have backgrounds of either crimi-
> nal behaviors or drug use, of course that's the same thing.

Nancy Foner, in *The Caregiving Dilemma* (1994), observed that while
bureaucratic rules often frustrate aides in nursing homes, such rules have a
role in preserving patient safety. Nursing homes, however, differ considerably from home settings in that there are few managers in home care to
enforce (or subtly subvert) bureaucratic rules. As a result, aides find themselves operating under a set of abstract bureaucratic constraints that seem
far removed from the realities of providing care in a home setting. The
most obvious bureaucratic shortsightedness stems from the fact that there
is often no one else to provide care to clients, especially if medical needs

arise suddenly. In these circumstances, aides feel compelled to act (by performing CPR, for example), but worry that such action might result in job loss or even a lawsuit. Virginia, a Maximum Care aide mentioned earlier, suggests that bureaucratic restrictions on care force aides to put the protection of self above the protection of clients. She describes the "line" aides must walk:

> I have to cover my company, I have to cover my butt. But I want to take care of my patients. You understand? So that's important. But I could be like some of them; I could walk in and say, "It's not my problem." Go home and leave. I'm not like that. You know, I just won't do it. And to my mind, any of these that do that, I just don't think that's right. But again, you're walking a fine line...you're only allowed to do so much.

Agonizing over the decision of whether to act or not to act in an emergency situation is a clear burden facing home care aides, but it is not one they face on a daily basis. Other bureaucratic norms, rules, and procedures, however, surface on a regular basis and, according to aides, detract from the quality of care they provide. Agencies certainly play a role in establishing and enforcing these rules, but regulations are also handed down from state and federal entitlement programs (such as the Medicaid waiver program) that restrict aides' scope of work. Without exception, aides interviewed serve a wide array of clients enrolled in publicly subsidized programs. Workers consequently have a great deal to say about the way that these programs limit both the emotional and physical work they can do. Beyond obvious restrictions on medical care, aides are generally prohibited from taking walks with clients, escorting patients to appointments, or simply taking them out for lunch or on an outing. Aides are not simply frustrated by the regulations; they find fault with an uneven application of the rules that appear contingent on the agency and type of insurance and/or benefits covering the client. Virginia, for example, has private-pay clients whom she regularly takes out to the park or to the doctor, sometimes just to "get fresh air." In other cases, however, Virginia is restricted from even taking a client for a walk around the block, unless she purchases her own liability insurance to do so.

Aides find the inconsistencies of these policies infuriating. Dot remembers a client who became eligible for Medicaid's Passport program, intended to provide personal care services to low-income elderly. Once her client enrolled in the program, Dot could no longer drive the client anywhere, which fundamentally disrupted their routine of five years, of driving each week to a nearby town to have lunch and get their hair done by one of the client's relatives. Dot expresses frustration that bureaucratic changes to client care fail to take into account the real needs of clients:

> This is ridiculous…at some point it's like you people need to go in the home and see exactly what these people need.…They've put so many guidelines on everything. I can understand the privacy, but then they come up with this HIPAA [Health Insurance Portability and Accountability Act]. With all this, I can't even discuss who I'm talking about to the receptionist because she's not allowed to know all this stuff. Some of those things are getting a little carried away.…Let's just say a lot of people, they need to go into these homes…have somebody go in and see what these people really need.

Dot goes on to say that bureaucratic restrictions on care, especially those that limit the ability of aides to draw on their soft skills and provide quality companionship, translate into a real loss for the relationship between caregiver and client:

> Even, you know, like going to doctor's appointments anymore, it seems like you have to have permission to go with them. It used to be either you took them or you got on the bus and you went with them, or whatever. I think something has been lost in that, because there are some people who need that. It's like one lady, she lived in Spring City. She lived there her whole life—she was eighty years old—she actually lived in the house that her grandparents built and she loved to just go driving around Spring City. I know more about Spring City.…She used to say, "Here is so-and-so's farm," and then we would go out to Johnson's farm and pick strawberries. To me, that is so much. For them to be able to get out and do stuff like that, especially when they have family that doesn't take them out. I think they lose a lot when they're just cooped up in the home.

It is important to say that, in contrast to aides working in nursing homes, home care aides face relatively few bureaucratic constraints. While the rules and regulations are there, enforcement of the rules appears uncommon, as aides often work independent of nurse or case managers.

Clients and, when present, their families, sometimes serve as a "check" on workers' behavior, but in the context of a strong aide-client bond, aides are generally left alone to consider rules and regulations. For the most part, aides in this study observe rules laid out by the agencies, especially those pertaining to restrictions on medical care. As Virginia and Dot show us, however, aides tend to question or ignore certain restrictions when they feel the client's health or emotional well-being is negatively impacted by bureaucratic dictates.

Agencies and For-Profit Care

Although some aides complain about the bureaucratic constraints associated with caregiving, almost all recognize that agencies have to demonstrate to clients and their families (as well as social service programs that pay for client care) that measures are in place to ensure safe, quality care. Aides are less forgiving, however, when it comes to what they regard as the for-profit logic of the agencies. As they see it, trying to increase the bottom line prevents agencies from acting in the best interests of clients and often leaves aides on the losing end of a moneymaking enterprise.

Patty, a white aide in her midthirties, works for a private home care agency in Ohio. Acknowledging that agencies are staffed by busy managers who have little time to perfect aide-client "matches," she nonetheless feels the agency rushes the process of pairing workers with clients in the interest of profit. The speed with which Patty was placed with her first client left her wondering about the agency's commitment to care:

> When I signed up, I went in, filled an application out, and I got names of clients. I didn't know—that's what I didn't like about it—I didn't know who they were, didn't know where they lived, I didn't know what kind of care was going to be needed when I went to the home. So when I went to each of my clients' houses, I was completely—I had no idea what I was going to walk into. I had no idea what was going to be needed.

Agencies are often just as quick to remove aides from client homes, sometimes with little or no warning and without clear reason (if, for example, the client requests the removal of an aide). For aides like Tammy, also in Ohio, it is both confusing and emotionally taxing to be "pulled" from a client with whom she has developed a bond or rapport over weeks or months. After one of her clients, a disabled elderly man, experienced a lapse in coverage, Tammy's agency eliminated the case from her roster. She was both concerned and saddened that the agency had terminated the relationship so abruptly:

> I go in there for six weeks, then I get a call, "You're not going there any-more." And then it's like, "Well do they know? Did you people call?" Be-cause this is a really nice family. I was raised in Middletown and they were raised in Greenville and...different things we did, and with his daugh-ter, and to some point you wonder what happens after you leave. After so long...it would have been nice to have a little bit of notice. Last week I could have said good-bye. I just get a phone call, "You're not going there anymore." So it's like, okay, I didn't get a chance. I'm disappointed.

Aides also identified agency practices that adversely affected their abil-ity to make a fair wage. Shelly, an aide in Ohio, previously worked for a large home care company with more than twenty-five franchises in the northern part of the state. The company asked Shelly to work seven days a week, promising her extra wages for working on her one day off a week. Reluctantly, Shelly agreed to work the full week, only to find later that she had not been compensated. After her manager denied offering her a pay increase for the work, Shelly left the company and vowed never to return to their agency again.

Unlike Shelly, other aides feel unable to walk away when agencies act unscrupulously. Kristen works for private-pay clients as well as for an agency in Middletown, Ohio. The agency is owned by two former nurse practitioners, who Kristen thinks reap the financial benefits of her labor while leaving little for her in terms of earnings. In need of work, Kris-ten feels trapped working for an agency that is, as she put it, "nickel-and-diming" her:

> I will stay with this. But do I like it? No. Do they think they've got some-thing cool going? You know, right? If they could sit and punch their thing, and make fifteen dollars, you know, it's sixty dollars a week. Both of them. And they get thirty people doing this, they're going to have a cool income. I'm going to be over here scrubbing and cleaning and, you know, laundry. That's what all these organizations do.

Generally speaking, aides working for IHSS complain less about un-scrupulous managers or unpaid wages and more about the bureaucratic way in which value (i.e., hours and wages) is assigned to their caregiving. Elderly and disabled clients who receive IHSS benefits are given a caseworker who assesses the needs of clients during a home visit (independent of the caregiver) and then allots a maximum number of hours for care. Some aides complain that elderly clients minimize their needs when talking to a caseworker, which can result in reduced hours and wages or, more commonly, a situation where an aide is underpaid for care. Workers feel they have little recourse when they aren't given enough hours for the work required, although some report making futile efforts to contact overworked and underpaid caseworkers. Common across all IHSS and private-agency workers is the belief that home care organizations—whether they are state run or privately run—put the needs of the organization before the needs of clients and workers. As a result, aides see themselves as relatively powerless against the for-profit or bureaucratic imperatives of home care agencies.

The Emotional Labor of Direct Care

Home care aides clearly perform a great deal of physical labor in the service of client care. Tasks like cleaning, bathing, grooming, feeding, and helping someone use the bathroom clearly involve a great deal of "body work" (Twigg 2000). Less obvious to the outside observer, however, is the degree of emotion work, or emotional labor, that aides provide to clients. Listening, talking, emoting, relating, counseling, reassuring, nurturing, coaxing, and arguing are all parts of an aide's job, although these "relational" aspects of the job often go unrecognized by agencies and policy-makers studying long-term care. As Maggie commented about the degree of emotional labor in her job, "Mentally, a caregiver is way underpaid. Sometimes you feel really unappreciated."

Sociologists studying other kinds of paid careworkers, such as nursing home assistants or nurses, have acknowledged the degree to which emotional labor structures the day-to-day work of caregivers, while also contributing to problems of burnout and turnover (Berdes and Eckert 2007; Erickson and Grove 2008; Lopez 2006). Home care aides differ considerably from caregivers working in institutional settings such as hospitals and nursing homes, however. Most obviously, home care aides provide care in the context of a private space, where the primary social relationship formed is between aide and client. While families may play a role in the setting, there are no co-workers, managers, or even other patients on-site. As such, the dyad of aide-client becomes central to the way that emotional labor is defined, carried out, and experienced by aides working in homes. This unique context of paid care has implications for the degree to which aides perceive emotional labor as taxing, draining, or tied to burnout.

To better understand why emotional labor differs by context (home versus institution), it helps to consider Hochschild's discussion of "feeling rules." As defined in her seminal work on emotion management (Hochschild 1979, 1983), "feeling rules are what guide emotion work by establishing the sense of entitlement or obligation that governs emotional exchanges....It is a way of describing how—as parents and children, wives and husbands, friends and lovers—we intervene in feelings in order to shape them" (1983, 56). While feeling rules certainly depend on the social actors involved (women and men have different relationships to feeling rules, for example) the context in which emotion work takes place is equally important to the construction of and adherence to feeling rules. For example, there are certain feeling rules at play when a woman cares for an ailing parent, namely, that she will express altruistic motivations for her care (rather than begrudging obligation) and will feel love and kindness toward her parent (rather than resentment or frustration). In contrast, paid caregivers who tend to the elderly in nursing homes must adhere to a different set of feeling rules, what Steve Lopez (2006) has identified as "organized emotional care," that contains elements of "detached politeness" as well as genuine affection toward patients. The bottom line, echoed by Lopez as well, is that the context of care influences how feeling rules are organized and experienced by social actors.

For home care aides, the context of care is somewhat complicated by social norms and feeling rules associated with both family and work. Workers, such as aides, who provide care or other services at the nexus of home and work prompt an exploration of emotional labor in what Hochschild identifies as "marketized private life," a third sector of social life that exists awkwardly between the realms of family and work (Hochschild 2003). Aides are not family in the formal sense of the word, but in many cases they end up providing care in ways that resemble familial care, preparing meals in a client's kitchen or playing cards while "visiting." The fact that caregiving takes place in the space of a home further reinforces the familial framing of the work, a reality that—as I discuss below—appears to affect aides' identity and emotional labor. Feeling rules in the context of home care seem to draw, not surprisingly, on social norms that emanate from the private space of home and family as well as the public space of work. At times this creates a sense of frustration for aides, who feel their status as pseudofamily leads to overwork, both emotionally and physically.

The titles, monikers, and labels that aides give themselves in reference to their work speak volumes about the complex social roles (and feeling rules) associated with caring for someone in the home. It is common for aides to give themselves familial titles—such as wife, mother, child, grandma, and friend—when characterizing their role in a client's home. Patty, for instance, calls herself "basically a wife" for the elderly man she works for four days a week, since she changes his bed and cleans the kitchen and bathroom. She goes on to say that after she's finished cleaning, she sits around and talks to him, about "gas prices and nothing." Virginia, sixty-two, says that after nearly thirty years of paid care work, her reputation—and the value she adds to the lives of others—precedes her. When I ask how she builds trust with her clients, she laughs me off, saying, "I'm like grandma. I'm little grandma in Ohio." And Tammy, fifty-one, compares her care of clients to a parent-child bond, replete with the attendant worries and concerns of parenthood: "But when I connect with someone,…it's very, very hard to disconnect, even temporarily. It's almost like having a child; you know the child's safe at school, and yet, you know there's always something in the back of your mind."

According to aides, agencies discourage workers from developing close bonds with clients, ostensibly to protect both sides of the dyad. As Dawn, from Ohio, explained, "We're supposed to have sympathy, not empathy, but anybody that's done this job very long is going to tell you, you get attached. You can't help it." Given how frequently aides' assignments change (and clients' lives change), there is good reason for the caution from agencies. Unlike aides working in nursing homes, where the routinization of care can preclude intense bonding with patients, home care aides can adhere to agency suggestions to maintain distance, or disregard these rules altogether. Most aides try to do a little of both: erect boundaries where possible, but not at the expense of cultivating companionship with clients. Walking an interactional line such as this is not easy for aides who spend hours a day in the informal space of a client's home. Finding a balance between establishing boundaries and developing connections is made easier when all parties—clients, aides, and agencies—recognize and tacitly agree on the feeling rules of the situation.

Tammy, whose relationship with her neighbor Sue was discussed earlier, believes that it is easier to construct and maintain emotional boundaries when clients acknowledge the need for them. As mentioned above, Tammy felt overwhelmed both emotionally and physically by her close ties to Sue, a problem exacerbated by the fact that Sue was an acquaintance before she was a patient. Tammy benefited emotionally from the close ties to Sue, but also felt strain from being in such close and constant proximity to her client. In other instances, Tammy has had better luck maintaining distance while caregiving. She explains:

> The agency says, in a very gentle way, "Try to maintain some sort of perspective on your client." And that's all they say. Most of these clients are accustomed to having new and strange people come into their house all the time. So they don't necessarily have an opportunity to form a kind of emotional attachment. So I think, partly, the clients help me with that unwittingly, and that they don't expect me to form an attachment. We haven't lived next door to each other. We haven't known each other's cats. [Current client] Maxine, she'll actually come out and say, "Should I not call you so much? I don't want to interfere." I mean, she's very aware that that's a danger. Sometimes she'll say, "Are you too involved with me?" And I can say, "No, dear, I'm not." I think she has been able to attach to me, and I haven't discouraged it. But I think she understands that I don't wholeheartedly, emotionally involve myself with her. I mean, it seems like a healthy partnering so far.

Tammy's story suggests that some clients (and aides) are aware that providing care in a home blurs boundaries in a way that could potentially lead to unhealthy emotional connections for both parties. Precisely because the domains of work and family are so blurred in home care, many caregivers and clients—like Tammy and Maxine—work consciously to negotiate the feeling rules associated with "marketized private life" (Hochschild 2003).

More commonly, however, aides and clients seem to differ (and sometimes conflict) in their respective understanding of feeling rules. This discrepancy surfaces when clients ask aides to take responsibility for tasks normally associated with the family, a problem that aides themselves often reinforce by describing their care and identity in familial terms, a subject I return to in greater detail in chapter 3. Recall Virginia, who sees herself as "a little grandma in Ohio." Although Virginia describes herself in this way without reservation, it angers and confuses her when she is asked to take on responsibilities customarily left to family or friends. Nonetheless, Virginia reports accepting additional work responsibilities, in part because she knows that clients do in fact see her as "family." She explains:

> I might be running, then they decide last minute they need something from the store. I've gone and done it, and, you know, come back [to the house]. . . . You know, they're like family after a while. You've been going to them. You know their most intimate part of their life because you're in their home and their body and their house, you know. So yeah, you do. You make extra things.

Virginia's sense of obligation to "make extra things" is clearly tied to complex (and contradictory) social rules cuing emotional engagement in this family/home/work setting. The intimate bonds that form between clients and caregivers in home care blur social roles for both sides of the dyad, which in turn confounds the rules of emotional exchange. Complex feeling rules can lead to situations where aides are unable or unwilling to draw clear boundaries with clients who, through no ill intent, seek additional help from a caregiver they have come to view as a close friend or family member.[2] While close ties to clients can be rewarding for aides, workers also experience very real stress managing the relational and emotional aspects of their job.

Stresses of Emotional Labor

Nearly all of the aides discussed in this book have a complex relationship to their emotional labor. For most caregivers, emotional labor is tied to both job satisfaction and a sense of burnout or fatigue. In what follows, I discuss four broad conditions under which emotional labor appears linked to negative psychosocial outcomes for caregivers: client stressors, family stressors, alienation, and surplus care. While I separate these categories for analytic purposes, aides generally experience some combination of these stressors at multiple points in their paid caring careers. The purpose here is not to demonstrate, causally, that certain conditions produce fatigue, burnout, or low job satisfaction. Rather, since the data here are ethnographic and interview-based, the discussion that follows is an attempt to provide descriptions of the range of emotional commitments that produce stress, as subjectively identified by aides themselves.

Client Stressors   For most aides, the daily reality of providing companionship and support to an elderly or disabled adult takes an emotional toll. This comes as no surprise, given the exhaustive literature that suggests that emotional labor can indeed have deleterious consequences for workers (Erickson and Wharton 1997; Hochschild 1983; A. Wharton 1999). One possible interpretation is that emotional labor encourages workers to "surface act," or perform, emotion in a way that contradicts their genuine emotional state ("service with a smile"). Hochschild and others argue that this type of emotion work can produce "emotive dissonance" and an alienation of the self (Ashforth and Humphrey 1993; Hochschild 1983; Leidner 1999; A. Wharton 1999). There are also negative consequences for workers when emotional labor produces a genuine overinvestment of the self into the well-being of others (Hochschild 1983). While I did find evidence to support the theory that aides sometimes "surface act" on the job in a way that produces burnout or fatigue, aides more commonly described unintended psychosocial consequences of "losing themselves" or overinvesting in client care. Even when aides have overwhelmingly positive relationships with clients, there is a degree of emotional fatigue that inevitably comes from the relational work of talking, listening, and emoting. Maggie, a veteran aide, sums it up this way: "Sometimes, they [the clients] tell the same thing over and over and over. But you sit there and listen. Physically, mentally, emotionally, it drains you after a while."

Aides often don't realize that they are experiencing a sense of fatigue or burnout from their work until their spouses or partners say something to them. Tammy, the aide who lived next door to a client, recalls coming home from a shift with Sue "emotionally exhausted":

> I think my husband is the one who clued me in to what was going on emotionally. One evening before bed he said, "You came home from Sue's at four thirty and you have not stopped talking about her." And I hadn't realized, so for six hours—that was a real wake-up call. To me that's not good. I mean, it's not healthy.

Although Tammy still works as an aide, she hopes to retrain as an accountant, since she has some experience keeping books for local businesses in Middletown (unlike most of the aides I met, Tammy has a bachelor's degree). Tammy indirectly cites emotional labor as a key factor in her decision to change her line of work, commenting, "I need to be a little less emotionally attached to those who are not in my immediate family."

Dot, on the other hand, sees herself working in home care indefinitely, but she is aware that attending to the emotional needs of clients takes a toll on her. Dot takes pride in the fact that she has close ties with many of her clients (recall her weekly excursions to the hairdresser with her elderly client), but she also recognizes that these "friendships" are a source of emotional strain for her:

> Like the client I have now, I mean, emotionally I know she's depressed. A lot of times I'm sitting there listening to her, and between her husband and the kid, it's like, I know! And sometimes when I leave it's just like, "Oh my goodness." It's just like, you feel drained. I mean, the work isn't hard; there's not a lot to do there. But emotionally it's like I know she needs something. Basically sometimes I feel like I'm more of a friend than actually her aide. Then some instances when you go there, the way the kids are, it can get to you sometimes.

Based on aides' accounts, it is clear that emotional fatigue or burnout is a regular, almost routine, occupational hazard associated with direct care. The data presented here cannot link such experiences to broader patterns of burnout and attrition of workers but do suggest that emotional labor is an intrinsic and inevitable part of the job. There are, however, those clients (or circumstances) that are by no means routine or normal and bring with them an unusual set of emotional strains for workers. These emotional stressors stem from the blurred physical and emotional boundaries characteristic of home care, which position aides in close proximity to clients' personal space and personal troubles. When a client is selling drugs out of her home, for example, or when a client regularly breaches personal boundaries by calling an aide at home in the middle of the night, the emotional labor involved in managing such situations exceeds the normal emotional "output" expected.

Dot, for example, cared previously for a housebound middle-aged client, Sadie, with debilitating arthritis. Sadie would call Dot nightly at home to demand a pack of cigarettes, which Sadie could not go out and buy herself. If Dot protested, as she did initially, then Sadie called incessantly until Dot changed her mind. Dot was aware that the client's behavior was unacceptable, but she stayed on the case for nearly a year, citing her gift for handling difficult clients. Those linked tangentially to the situation, including Dot's husband and the visiting nurses working the case, found the client intolerable. Dot concurred with their assessment, but also took pride in the fact that she could handle a client who had alienated all others around her:

> [My husband] wanted me to quit. He said, "You need to quit this. Go to Walmart. You need to get out of this." It was just so frustrating. I even had nurses that quit going to her.... One nurse said, "I had to go down the street and park for fifteen minutes before I go to my next client, to calm down." She said, "I don't know how you do this."

Dot cited Sadie's "situation at home," specifically her verbally abusive son, as one of the reasons she stayed as long as she did. Despite Dot's willingness to work with such a client, the emotional labor involved in caring for a demanding person took a clear toll on Dot's psyche. After her husband routinely complained that she was "a bear" when she got home from a shift, Dot quit and then moved with her husband to California for six months. On returning to Ohio, Dot was asked by her agency to once again assume care of Sadie. Dot refused, and later found out that Sadie had gone through seven or eight agencies before coming back to the first, desperate to find a caregiver. Sadie continues to call Dot for favors and to beg her to come back into her home. Dot is not tempted in the slightest, telling me, "I did more for her than anybody else will, but I told [the agency], there's no way."

Other clients have life circumstances—tied to the realities of poverty, addiction, depression, or mental illness—that make the work of caregiving taxing at best. Shelly has worked for a handful of clients who are heavy users of drugs or alcohol. One of these clients, Tawna, is a middle-aged white woman who lives "back in the woods," which is how Shelly describes clients who live in the rural areas surrounding Middletown. When Shelly took the case, the agency briefed her about the problem, assuring her that Tawna, identified as an alcoholic, was now in recovery. Shelly soon discovered otherwise, finding a crack pipe in the woman's bedroom during a routine cleaning of the house. Shelly reported the problem to the case manager at the agency, who did nothing to alter the situation. After "living with it" for nearly a month, Shelly demanded reassignment, a request the agency eventually granted. Shelly explains:

> You can only do so much before you're like, "No. Enough." And the unfortunate part is I adore that woman. But I will not go over there and watch her kill herself, because it would be one thing if she was doing something that was a little more herbal, that people don't die from overdosing on. But, you know, I'm pretty sure what I found wasn't herbal.

Patty, in Central City, has never encountered drug addiction in her clients, but she has experienced stress as a result of caring for a client, Callie, who is severely mentally and physically handicapped. Callie is a disabled woman in her fifties, a former college professor left paralyzed and mentally impaired by a serious car accident that occurred in her forties. Patty finds it challenging to interact with Callie, since she has both short- and long-term memory loss (Callie often forgets who Patty is between visits, and Patty must spend time each visit reminding Callie of her family members' names and whereabouts). Callie is mentally ill as a result of her brain injury, and suffers from obsessive-compulsive disorder. As Patty tells it, Callie's illness manifests as compulsive interests in foods (she eats only marshmallows) and an obsession with both suicide and death. Even though Callie's doctors assure Patty that these macabre interests are unlikely to lead Callie to harm herself, Patty still feels the stress of trying to relate to a client who talks regularly about such alarming topics. Patty explains:

> I do listen to her [Callie]. And then there's been times where I'm like, "Okay. You're scaring me. Are you really going to do something like this? Do I need to take you to go to the [doctor]…?" She'll say, "Oh no, I'm fine." But, you know, there's been a couple times where I'm like, "You're really scaring

me." Or, you know, "You don't want to just wipe yourself off the face of the earth. What is your mom going to do? What's your family going to do? You know, you're here by yourself; how would anybody know? I don't want to come and find you some Tuesday laying on your bed dead." [Callie says,] "Oh no, you don't have to worry about that. It's nothing like that." But there's been times where…you know, I don't know what I'm going to walk into on Tuesday.

Patty expresses deep sympathy for Callie's situation and finds many aspects of the caregiving relationship truly rewarding. Callie, for example, remains an accomplished ceramics artist despite her illness and spends time teaching Patty how to work with clay on a pottery wheel. Nonetheless, Patty finds herself worrying about her client's well-being "after hours," a reality that she finds unsettling and emotionally taxing.

Managing client behavior, such as drug use or mental illness, is an unanticipated part of the job that can produce workplace strain for aides. Some stresses, however, are anticipated by both agencies and aides and viewed as a natural part of the job. Specifically, aides enter home care with an acute awareness that they will likely care for people at the end of life and witness one or more client deaths. Most aides do not predict, however, the emotional stress of caring for someone experiencing a painful or prolonged death trajectory. Tammy, recounting her experiences with her client (and neighbor) Sue, explained that watching her suffer through extreme pain at the end of life was an emotionally difficult and demanding part of the job. Tammy was not merely a witness to Sue's decline but a key participant in the complex interpersonal dynamics that form when a care recipient is severely depressed, in pain, or nearing death. Tammy explains:

I loved her so much. We were just so close. And honestly it was like knowing my sister was in pain, all the time, and there was so little, really so little that I could do. So I think that just became really just part of my life, my daily life, and my emotional life. When I started feeling in deep water I think was about the last year of her life. Her pain levels increased so much. She was medicated of course, and under a doctor's care. But I found that we were so close that she was able to really express what she was going through. And it was not positive at all. So our relationship kind of started changing then; I became more of a—hmm, what's the word I want? More of a motivator for her. And sometimes that took the form of, you know, I had to be very firm with her and even pretend to get angry at times, which she saw through, but she still accepted that. It was a very complex situation. I just learned so much about her and myself and her family and how to integrate all those experiences.

Maggie experiences similar feelings when she witnesses her clients in intense pain, generally at the end stages of life:

> In the beginning it's not bad. It's just as time progresses, it's so sad to watch somebody brilliant all of the sudden just go downhill to like nothing practically. It breaks my heart. You want to do something. There's nothing you can do except be kind to them…and make them as comfortable as possible.

Agencies prepare aides for the inevitability of client death and encourage strict emotion rules to prevent extended feelings of grief ("don't get attached"; "don't become a friend"), but most aides find these distancing techniques difficult to practice, especially with clients to whom they have a strong tie. As a result, aides often experience intense emotions when a client passes. José, a Puerto Rican aide in his fifties, explains how he feels when a client dies:

> You get close to people, you know. First thing they taught me when I was in school was, don't get attached. And I said, "Oh well." But it's a lot of malarkey; it doesn't work that way, not in real life. You could tell somebody that, but when you're working, you know, you get close to somebody, and when that person passes on, you feel it. They say that it gets easier, you know, to accept, but every once in a while you're going to have someone who's special to you and it's going to hurt.

Dawn has experienced roughly five client deaths in her tenure as an aide. Recently, Dawn showed up for her daily shift with an elderly client, Eva, and found that she had died hours earlier. Dawn was traumatized by the fact that Eva had clearly died only a short time before her arrival ("She'd been expecting us; she was still warm"). When I asked Dawn to describe Eva's death, it became clear that it was not the grief per se that created emotional strain, but rather her agency's decision to downplay and ignore her feelings of loss.

The last supervisor I had at [the agency], she didn't understand the connection. She did not understand that we got attached to these people no matter what. She just didn't get it. She'd never done it.... I was made to work the rest of the day. I was made to work. [Taking part of the day off] was not an option. I was not supposed to grieve my patient. I was not supposed to be that attached. [It] didn't matter that I took care of her for two and a half years, that she was frail and didn't have anybody really.... She [the supervisor] didn't even bother to call and say, "Eva's gone."

Dawn's account is an example of how agencies promote "disenfranchised grief" among aides (Doka 1989) by denying them access to socially sanctioned and publicly shared rituals of grief (taking time off work, openly mourning, etc.). So even though aides often form family-like bonds with clients, these informal connections are not always recognized by others, such as agency supervisors or biological family members. Since agencies generally instruct aides to erect clear emotional boundaries (again, enforcing a set of bureaucratically driven feeling rules), experiencing multiple client deaths can take a toll on aides who are doubly burdened by both the psychological dimensions of grief and the agency's bureaucratic dictates to "move on." For this reason, some aides—like Dawn—directly link client deaths to their own feelings of burnout:

I actually dropped out of the field for a couple of years. Because the burnout at that point was, I mean, I buried a lot of patients, and it gets to you. When you do this job right, you leave a little piece of yourself with everyone you encounter, and it gets to the point where you can't leave them anymore.

Relationships with Families   When an aide secures a job working in a client's home, she generally considers the client to be her employer, with the agency playing an important, albeit distant, secondary role. In many instances, however, the client's family is part of the picture, serving to both enhance and complicate aides' caregiving. As discussed earlier, families often openly embrace aides, inviting them to family events, dinners, and outings. While this can overburden aides, being "part of the family" or a fictive family member also helps reinforce job satisfaction and identity formation on the job.

Family life, however, is not always rosy, a fact that bears directly on the life experiences of clients and the work experiences of aides. Aides expend emotional labor helping clients manage their families, usually in those circumstances when family members (a spouse, a daughter or son) are absent or negligent, or when they try to dictate the organization of care from afar. In addition, tumultuous home life can make an aide's job exceptionally difficult, especially in terms of the emotional energy she must use to care for a client in such a context.

Aides are often frustrated by families who they perceive as negligent in their care of a relative, especially when those families live nearby and appear to have the kind of resources—time and money—that would allow for greater involvement. Virginia cares for an elderly client, Edith, who lives alone on the outskirts of Middletown. Edith's family lives a short drive away, but they generally leave her alone in conditions that Virginia feels are less than safe. Virginia is with Edith four or five hours a day, but the elderly woman otherwise manages her dementia and frequent epileptic episodes alone. Virginia has noticed that the smoke detectors in the home don't work; that there are no flashlights or other emergency aides should Edith need them; and that parts of the house are impassable because the family chooses to store boxes and miscellaneous furniture in Edith's home. When the family went on vacation, Virginia was "heartbroke" out of fear that Edith would hurt herself and have no family to call. Virginia decided to stop in and check on Edith, outside of her designated hours. In her assessment, the family left for vacation with little forethought about the difficulties Edith might face as a result:

> They took off, nobody was checking on her. Her medication, they gave her a box she couldn't get open. They got her a brand-new one, then she couldn't open it because her hands are going bad. I mean, I was just—And even her visiting nurse, he just said, "This is ridiculous." I'm like, "Well, one day she'll overdose and we'll find her dead." And that'll be my present to me, that I get to find her like that, you know. Those things bother me. I try not to dwell on them. I let her call me. They're not supposed to have our phone number, but I let her call me.

When I ask Virginia whether Edith calls regularly, even when the family is in town, she replies, "Yeah. She'll call me. She'll say, 'Please call me back.'

And she'll tell me what's going on. But I try to call her back, if not immediately, quick, you know. Sometimes she just wants to gab. She wants somebody. And they live right there."

As de facto advocates, aides can become sounding boards for clients experiencing family dysfunction. Tammy sees this as part of the job, even though family tumult induces personal stress:

> I have had clients, a couple of clients, that had no family involvement whatsoever. Very bad times with their family. And it was just vitriolic. I would get the anger and all that hurt, you know, all those stories, "he said, she said." And that's part of care. You know, it's not always pleasant, but it's part of it.

When clients live with family, aides often witness unhealthy family dynamics firsthand. Dot takes care of a client in her early sixties who is recovering from extensive surgery to remove part of her colon after doctors discovered she had "massive blood clots." According to Dot, the client, Kath, is very weak, wears a colostomy bag, and requires direct care most of her waking hours. Her quality of life will improve once she receives additional surgery, but Dot is unsure when this will happen. Dot considers Kath a "friend," but has a difficult time managing the relationship because Kath's "home situation isn't good." Kath's husband neglects his caregiving role, leaving most of the work to Dot during her four- or five-hour shift. Other family members in Kath's home also negatively affect her well-being and mental health, something that by extension makes Dot's job more difficult:

> It makes it hard because I'd like to take her husband and smack him upside the head. And her son, some of the things he does....It's kind of difficult but I'd never leave her....I think I'm really her sounding board. There are times, it's just like, "Okay, you know, what can I do about it?" But I know she needs to talk about it....I would say she's clinically depressed.

Whether managing family dysfunction or filling in the "care gap" left by negligent family members, some aides are unequivocal about the challenges of working with clients' families. Shelly says, "I can't stress enough, dealing with [families] is worse than dealing with the patients. Because they have these high expectations. There are times that I'm just like, why am I doing this?" Reiterating a second time that "the worst part of the job is dealing with the families," Shelly tells me about one of her "ladies," Polly, an elderly woman with dementia whose family presents problems. In Shelly's view, the family insists on organizing Polly's care in a certain way even though they lack an understanding of Polly's day-to-day needs. Shelly told me of a recent incident where she alerted the family to a problem with Polly's medication:

> [I told them], "Your mother has dementia. She's not taking her pills." [Polly] has this awesome med machine, and when the meds come down, it says, "It's time to take your meds, Polly." But Polly hides them under her chair. So when I try to run this past the daughter and the granddaughter and, you know, even the agency, [they say,] "Well, she has a machine that reminds her." Well, doesn't matter, it scares her. I mean, I'm sorry, if something was talking to me and said my name, I might be a little creeped out too. But people don't understand that the worst part of this job is not the stuff we have to do for [the clients] because their family's not doing it—it's the family. Dealing, coping with their problems. Not so much the rest of us, or the patients.

Shelly concludes that "family shouldn't be as involved with the aides. I shouldn't have to report to them. I don't work for the family; I work for the residents and I work for a company. I mainly work for the company.... That is such a big stress, when you put ten different people in the mix." Shelly obviously has strong views on the issue of family involvement, likely stemming from her negative experiences dealing with Polly's family. Shelly's frustration notwithstanding, one can imagine scenarios where being a "meddlesome" or micromanaging family member is necessary in order to preserve the safety and well-being of a loved one. Although aides in this study, by all accounts, approach their work conscientiously, the problem of substandard care is a real one. Aides understand this and express disdain for "other" paid caregivers in the field who sully the reputation of the group. The point here is not to resolve whether family behavior is defensible or aides' irritation justified, but to understand that the management of families on an interpersonal level is a very real part of paid care work and, as such, constitutes a significant part of the emotional labor expended. Meanwhile, it is important to note that aides do not view families in an entirely negative light. As I discuss in chapter 3, aides frequently cite fictive family ties to clients and their clients' families as a central *reward* of paid care work. Families, as such, have the potential both to enhance and to detract from workers' overall sense of job satisfaction.

Alienation   There are moments when the job of being an aide produces a sense of alienation, akin to that which is described by Hochschild and other scholars studying emotional labor in service work (Erickson and Wharton 1997; Hochschild 1983; Leidner 1999; Macdonald and Sirianni 1996; Wharton 1999). Similar to the flight attendants described by Hochschild (1983) and the fast-food workers in Leidner's (1993, 1999) studies, aides describe feeling constrained, unfulfilled, or demeaned by the more routine aspects of the job, particularly cleaning. In addition, aides occasionally take direct verbal abuse from clients, which, not surprisingly, contributes to feelings of alienation. Alienation appears to be most acute when client behaviors or actions directly call into question aides' sense of self on the job. Specifically, aides view themselves as offering comprehensive care to clients that includes both physical and emotional components. When clients reduce aides' work to the physical aspects of the job, openly referring to them as "maids," for example, feelings of alienation can ensue.

Virginia links feelings of alienation to changes in her scope of work, which limits the amount of hands-on care she can provide clients. Speaking about an elderly client whom she sees regularly, Virginia comments:

> It's now doing general cleaning. I mean, that's all I do. I've never laid a hand on this guy....I don't cook for him. All I do is go in and clean. I'm the cleaning lady, you know. And that's kind of how they think of you. That's probably my biggest complaint, is I just clean.

Virginia adds that she cleans for other family members in addition to the client, doing laundry or dishes for his daughter and grandchildren who visit frequently (she recalls arriving one day to find fifteen loads of laundry that the family had dropped off for her to do). Aides are particularly resentful of those clients who are mobile, active, and socially engaged and treat home care as a housecleaning service. Patty expressed her frustration in this way, referring to an elderly client for whom she works:

> She's got a very large core of friends. And she stays active, and she goes out to places, stuff like that. I guess for her I'd say I'm just a glorified maid. I'll walk in sometimes and there's dirty dishes everywhere in the kitchen. And my mind-set is, "Okay. I'm sure that you could wash some of these dishes." But it seems like—and I don't want to sound negative, but it seems like she really leaves everything that has to be done for when I come....She don't have to do anything. Yeah, I have a week's worth of dishes, and then I have three loads of laundry, and I do her bathroom, and I vacuum, and sweep, and mop.

Simply put, doing more cleaning than caring leads some aides to feel alienated from their professional work, their "calling." Usually these "cleaning-heavy" cases are balanced with those that require more hands-on care or interactive emotion work, providing aides with sufficient opportunities to foster meaningful attachments to work. When client behavior is the source of aides' alienation, however, the negative feelings can be powerful and long lasting. Shelly described feelings of intense humiliation after she spent a day working for a new client, a young paraplegic man. When she was five minutes late to her first shift, the client "cursed and cursed" Shelly's tardiness, and then proceeded to mock her as she struggled through her first work task, brushing his teeth. Raw emotions apparent, Shelly remembered how the encounter made her feel: "I went one time. And it was an hour. And it felt like seven hours. I wanted to cry or burn the house down. It was sickening. It was sickening. But, you know, it's just how some people are.... And people like that, there's no hope. It was bad."

Lete, working in Central City, California, also experiences a certain degree of humiliation at work. Unlike Shelly, however, Lete remains committed to her client. Lete's client Mavis, an elderly white woman, constantly nags at Lete, telling her that she is "fat" and that she eats too much junk food. When Mavis goes to the doctor, with Lete's help, Mavis makes Lete wait in the car because she doesn't want Lete talking with the doctors and nurses. In recounting her story, Lete grew noticeably emotional, saying "sometimes she [Mavis] looks at me like I'm an enemy." Mavis cautions Lete that she is keeping an eye on her, making sure Lete does not steal anything. "I know how you are," Mavis tells Lete. Because of these tensions, Lete describes a relationship to her client that vacillates between care and contempt. Summing up their bond, Lete says, "Sometimes I feel so close to her; other times she totally changes."

As Lete's story illustrates, there are times when aides feel dehumanized by clients. Or as Maggie puts it, "People feel like they own you." Similarly, Andrew, an aide living in California, expresses frustration about his client's relentless and unrealistic demands:

> Sometimes he [the client] comes in with a big demand, you know, and he forgets that I'm human; he thinks I'm a robot. Like I say, it has to take a special type of person to do this kind of work because, you know, sometimes people, clients, they forget that you're human. They don't care. You have to remind them that, "Hey, look, I'm a human being."

Andrew's response when his clients treat him this way is to plainly explain to them how their behaviors belittle him. Although it may be difficult to imagine such an honest exchange, it makes sense when the complex power relations between clients and aides are taken into consideration. As several anecdotes in the chapter illustrate, there are times when clients assert that they are "in charge," a reality that can lead to feelings of alienation among aides. These feelings of alienation are tempered by two mediating factors that allow aides to maintain their own sense of self respect in the interaction. First, clients are often frail or disabled and unable to carry out their daily activities without the assistance of another person. Highly dependent on an aide to eat, go to the bathroom, or move around, clients must consider their behavior carefully. This is not to say that clients avoid all conflict (nor should they), but that there is a certain loss of power for dependent elderly or disabled adults who rely on paid caregivers for assistance. Second, unlike caregivers working in nursing homes, aides who experience verbally abusive situations in home-based care—as Shelly did—generally ask for a case reassignment. While these requests are not always granted, aides know that there are more clients in need of care than there are caregivers, which gives them some power with respect to both the agency and the client. Because of this, extreme feelings of alienation appear to be the exception, not the rule, for aides.

Surplus Care   Looking beyond the problem of worker alienation, there is another troubling way in which occupational inequality manifests in home care. Specifically, aides are often pressured—by clients, by agencies, and by themselves—to go "above and beyond." Aides who have close bonds with clients over extended periods of time can find themselves in situations where they are being asked to stay a little longer for dinner, lend a little money, or take on a little more cooking and cleaning beyond the terms of their contract. I call this extra labor performed by aides "surplus care."

The problem of surplus care is exacerbated by procedures of remuneration. Although the client constitutes a kind of "boss," or employer, if an aide is employed by an agency, then the client does not directly compensate an aide for services; it is the agency that sets the hours and wages and coordinates payroll. This commercial exchange for care is largely invisible to the client, further blurring the line between informal and formal labor already present in home-based care work (Folbre 2001; Harrington Meyer 2000). In this context, norms of interaction, or feeling rules, become somewhat confused (Are we family? Are we employer and employee?), such that aides feel obligated to provide for clients in ways that extend beyond their formal work commitments. As Rosa put it when I asked her to describe her work tasks: "We're maids plus, you know? Maids plus companion, maids plus nurse, maids plus family."

Virginia, from Middletown, recalls one Christmas holiday when a long-time client, Maxine, asked her in desperation to come in an extra day to help bake pies for out-of-town family coming to stay:

> I mean, they wanted me to bake ten pies for them. Sometimes they just get a little bit off, and if you don't know how to deal with that—I told you how long it's been I've been doing this; I better be able to handle it, you know? I was so frustrated when it came time to do all that [baking]. I mean, right up on the holiday day, you know, the day before, when everybody was there, I helped to get the things ready. And I said, "Oh, please don't do that to me next year." But you do it, you do it. They're good people. And there are some people that'll take advantage of you. And you have to be strong enough to say, "Hey," you know, "not a good thing. Let's think about something else." Sometimes you do have to learn how to say no.

Virginia felt "taken advantage of" by her client and, to be sure, there is an element of exploitation in the situation. But how did it come to this? Virginia talked earlier in the interview about feeling a close bond to Maxine, but believing nonetheless that the client "crossed the line" on this occasion. Idiosyncrasies of the individual client notwithstanding, such conflicts can also be understood as a by-product of confused feeling rules in the setting. Is Virginia a daughter to elderly Maxine? Is she a friend? Or is she a paid worker? Of course, she is all these things to Maxine, with the result that feeling rules associated with all these roles are operating in the setting.

At times, clients can be very blunt or emotionally manipulative when they want aides to go above and beyond for them. Sophie, an aide who recently immigrated to Central City from Hungary, was essentially "guilted" into forgoing her own family holiday commitments to satisfy the needs of her client.

> Now in this family, they made me kind of part of the family, and the lady was very nice, but, with being part of the family, they expected me to be with her when the daughter was out of town on Thanksgiving. I said, "Well, I would like to visit my husband's family in Southern California." She said, "Well, I will need you because my daughter's out of town and I need you."

Even when aides resist client guilt trips, they sometimes feel emotionally burdened by the regret or guilt of not giving more time. Mary, sixty-seven, tells me that she feels guilty that she doesn't do enough for her client, Antonia:

> Sometimes I think she thinks I'm not doing my share. I mean, I get this feeling. But she never says anything to me about it because, I mean, we have a good rapport. But then I feel a little guilty about that, you know, like I should probably be doing more and that maybe she kind of expects me to, but doesn't ask me to.

As is the case for the domestics discussed in Hondagneu-Sotelo's *Domestica* (2001), the rhetoric and logic of the "family bond" in home care masks the inequality and exploitation of the care work arrangement. Kelly, a white sixty-year-old aide, often lets her client sleep at her home, even though the terms of their contract forbid this. Kelly is paid for three hours of care a day but often spends a week of uninterrupted time with her elderly client. She is aware of breaking the rules, but says that both she and the client like the companionship and that the client is afraid to stay alone at night in her home. Kelly tells me: "It's not an issue. We're friends. We enjoy each other's company and we go out to eat together. I'm on Section 8 and don't have much rent to pay, so I don't need a whole lot of money."

On occasion, the costs of surplus care *are* financial. Given that many of the clients they care for are also poor (either poor to begin with or poor because they've "spent down" their savings in order to qualify for Medicare and/or Medicaid coverage), aides sometimes help cover expenses that the client can't manage alone. Martina, a fifty-seven-year-old African American aide, recounts a story about paying for her client's medication because it was no longer covered by insurance:

> A lot of medicines, you can only get seven prescriptions a month, and when we went to the neurologist, the neurologist said, "Well, I'm going to give you some lidocaine pads." He gave me the prescription, and I went to the pharmacist, and the pharmacist said, "They're not going to pay for this." I said, "Okay, how much is it?" They were $175. So what are you going to do? Then after I bought them and we put them on his foot...he said it froze it and he didn't like it, and it didn't help, so now I'm stuck with $175 worth of lidocaine pads. And the Vicodin he takes, Medi-Cal doesn't pay for them because they're too strong, but it doesn't matter anymore because he won't take them, but those I paid $78 for.

Shelly also pays for a few things here and there, explaining that it is difficult to avoid small acts of charity when a client is in need:

> I go above and beyond. If somebody needs something from the drugstore, and I can do it without breaking my wallet, and they don't have the money, sometimes I do that. And I would probably get fired if they found that out. But you can only watch somebody go without something for so long, that they really want or really need.

Although Shelly does reach into her own pocket for things her clients need (this despite her own reliance on public assistance to make ends meet), she draws clearer boundaries around other forms of surplus care, namely, visiting or communicating with clients after work hours. For example, Shelly was asked on two occasions by a client to come over for Sunday dinner and she refused flatly, with little remorse. She explains, "I love all those people to death. I love them very much. Unfortunately, I can't lose my job to make someone else feel better." It is not uncommon for aides to have quite rigid boundaries about some things that they perceive to be beyond their work duties, while simultaneously allowing for others (like paying for items that clients want or need).

Andrew is another aide who absorbs some of the costs associated with his client's care. The client is a young, mentally ill man "living in" with Andrew and his wife because he requires full supervision. Andrew's contract specifies that the client must pay him over five hundred dollars for rent, although when I interviewed Andrew, he had recently relaxed the terms of the contract. Even though Andrew only recently secured enough paid hours a month for the care of his client, he still willingly subsidizes the client's rent:

> At first I was getting ninety-something [hours per month], now I get 132. And I never get a day off. Every day I have to do something for him, morning, noon, and evening. In the agreement he pays me rent for staying here. He's not a big eater. I provide him with two meals per day, and that's including his rent and utilities, and I'm pretty fair because at first the rent was like $550, and for him I was seeing that he was struggling with that, he was having real problems, so I dropped it all the way from that to four hundred dollars. That's including everything.

While Andrew's paid hours have been "upped" to near full-time, he hints that this is not enough compensation, given that he provides full care. The larger question is why someone like Andrew, as a low-income caregiver, is absorbing financial responsibility for a client whose federal disability allowance fails to even cover his rent. Once Andrew's client had settled into his home, it became difficult for Andrew to remain rigid about the terms of the work contract, an example of the way that the blurred boundary between formal and informal labor helps sustain surplus care (we will learn more about Andrew's arrangement with his live-in client in chapter 3).

When aides are asked to give a little more on the job, stay a little longer, or provide financial or even emotional support long term, their care work generates surplus care from which agencies and clients benefit, at least in the short term. Workers themselves, while aware that the terms of the arrangement are not necessarily fair, willingly take on the extra work because of the benefits that home care work affords them relative to other kinds of service work, but also because they invest in the welfare of a client over time and cannot easily extract themselves from a potentially exploitative arrangement.

Agencies, who get a great deal of labor out of their employees at relatively little expense, also profit from the surplus care generated by aides who are willing to go "above and beyond." The problem, however, goes beyond individual caregivers and their employers. A lack of social support for the long-term care needs of the chronically ill and disabled in the United States—not to mention the lack of support for caregivers—means that governments, managed care organizations, hospitals, and even individual families all benefit from the surplus care provided by aides. While many aides are willing to insist on a high ethic of care, even without fair remuneration, the surplus care often comes at their emotional and financial expense.

The accounts offered here suggest that, in addition to the surplus labor of paid caregiving, aides find their work physically and emotionally taxing, at least some of the time. Aides are also frustrated by low wages and the poverty conditions of their lives, inconsistent hours and unpredictable work schedules, lack of training, and the imposition of bureaucratic rules and procedures by agencies. These findings help contextualize the problems of burnout and turnover so often discussed in the literature on long-term care and reaffirm that the constraints of low-waged care work can negatively affect aides' job satisfaction and well-being.

Given these very real constraints, why do workers choose home care? And why do they stay? In the second half of the book, I consider factors that compel many women, and some men, to take on low-waged care work, even in the face of structural disadvantage. While limited opportunity partially explains why women and men end up working in the field of home care, this lack of choice is not central to aides' own work narratives. Caregivers involved in the study are sometimes critical of the everyday inequalities of paid care work but in general emphasize that the job is personally rewarding, affords them a degree of autonomy, and imparts a sense of dignity not often found in the service sector. What is sociologically relevant, then, is the way in which aides construct an affirming workplace identity—what I call the caring self—in the context of occupational disadvantage.

3

The Rewards of Caring

ANDREW

While attending a series of on-the-job training courses for home care aides, I met Andrew, an aide living and working in Central City, California. Andrew was an eager participant in the training sessions and appeared, at times, to have more firsthand knowledge of the subject matter than the registered nurses leading the courses on "Universal Precautions" and "Personal Care for Your Client." After I made an announcement during a break about my study and the need for interview subjects, Andrew approached me to express interest in the research. I asked whether he would like to meet at his place of work or if he preferred to meet off-site. Andrew paused and told me to meet him at his house, and then added, "Which is where I work." We agreed to meet up midafternoon the following day.

Andrew owns a ranch-style home in a mixed-income suburb of Central City, an area populated predominantly by working-class Asian American and African American families. I greeted Andrew in the driveway as he returned from visiting the homes of his five regular clients. Initially confused by Andrew's comment that he worked at home, I realized after entering the front door and seeing miscellaneous medical paraphernalia that one of Andrew's clients lived with him. I learned that Andrew shared his home with two people: his wife of twenty years, and Rusty, a white male quadriplegic in his early forties who became paralyzed four years earlier as the result of a suicide attempt. After his accident, Rusty applied for support from IHSS in the hope of finding an aide to provide home-based care (Rusty was being discharged from a four-year stay at a convalescent hospital). After IHSS "matched" Andrew and Rusty, Andrew learned of his new client's need for housing and offered to rent him a room for below-market rates.

For Andrew, providing around-the-clock care to another person was in no way unusual. Caring first for his disabled mother and later, after she died, his developmentally delayed brother, Andrew had spent the last twenty years looking after chronically ill family members. Andrew's brother, Tim, passed away roughly a year prior to our interview, and Andrew was still visibly shaken by the loss. Although Tim had had ongoing problems with his kidneys, lungs, and heart, he died rather unexpectedly after doctors performed emergency surgery for an obstruction of the stomach. Andrew describes his psychological state after losing his brother:

> After my brother passed away, you know, it was kind of like a psychological impact. I needed income, I was going through a mental thing. I mean, that was my brother. After two years like that—I seen him suffer for the last two years. I still have a problem with that now, and then all of a sudden he just up and died and I had all my time. After, you know, twenty-four hours, seven days a week working with him, taking him places, taking him out for entertainment.

Andrew felt the grief following Tim's death acutely, and within a few months of the funeral he placed several ads in the paper advertising his services as an aide. With years of experience caring for family and non-relatives in nursing homes, Andrew easily secured four clients through a private agency, and then eventually found Rusty through IHSS. When I asked Andrew why he jumped into paid caregiving so quickly after his brother's death, he responded, "It's like I had to be caring for something, I don't care if it's the plant. I have to care for something. This is

in me, you know?" Although Rusty is gradually becoming more independent, Andrew spends most of his "at-home" time providing companionship to Rusty, who Andrew characterizes as "institutionalized,"
referring to his tendencies to withdraw from human interaction.

From time to time Andrew entertains the idea of finding work outside of caregiving (he has worked in a welfare office, as a telemarketer,
and as a security guard) and ultimately wants to get a license in real
estate. The lack of pay is a significant drawback of the job for Andrew,
who tells me, "They [the agencies] don't pay me enough for what I do."
Although Andrew's wife has a good desk job working for the state, he is
frustrated that his wages constitute a meager portion of the household
income. Andrew is also concerned that his body has been irreversibly
damaged by his care work, even though he admits that others find this
hard to believe since he is a large, muscular man who stands well over
six feet tall. Last year, a male client also over six feet and weighing 250
pounds fell on Andrew's left hip, aggravating an injury he had sustained
fifteen years ago when he "caught" another male client made unstable
by his Parkinson's. In addition to the injuries, Andrew experiences occa-
sional mistreatment by agencies and some clients.

Recently, Andrew was called out to the home of a wealthy, elderly
white woman with multiple sclerosis who needed to be transferred
(moved from bed to wheelchair) so that she could be cleaned and her
necrotic tissue disinfected. The woman's regular aide, a small woman,
could not lift her client, so the agency asked Andrew to fill in for the
day. Andrew was hoping to make some extra money moving and tending to the client, but when he arrived, he soon realized that his only
task was to move the very frail patient. The agency told Andrew not
to look at the woman's body as he transferred her, as the client feared
being touched by a male aide. The transfer took nearly an hour and the
woman shrieked insults at Andrew each time he touched her. Although
Andrew understood that the woman was in pain, he felt she had unrea-
sonable expectations that he act like "Hercules." Adding insult to injury,
Andrew was never compensated by the agency for his time.

Even though the low pay and intermittent moments of alienation give Andrew pause about his job, he remains tied to paid care work for the fore-
seeable future. The question is, why? The most obvious answer is that
Andrew is structurally positioned to do so, given his limited education and

job skills, physical impairments, age, race, and history of providing informal care to family. For an African American man in his fifties who has spent much of his life caring for family, nursing aide is part of a predictable "career line" (Spenner, Otto, and Call 1982). Another possible reason, put forth by economist Candace Howes, is that working as a home care aide is in fact a "good enough" job relative to other unskilled jobs in the service sector (Howes 2005). Howes points out that wages and benefits have slowly improved for aides, especially in states like California or New York where unions have organized workers. Andrew may be one of the many aides who remain in their line of work because the job is, simply put, good enough.

Although there are clear economic motivators—wages and benefits— that drive the recruitment and retention of aides, survey data on home care workers in California suggest other psychosocial factors also at play (Howes 2008). Sampling 2,260 home care workers employed by IHSS in California, Howes (2008) finds that "commitment to consumer" is the most common reason aides cite for taking a job in home care, regardless of wage levels or personal characteristics. Curiously, even though her own data indicate that there are clear nonmaterial motivations propelling women and men into paid care work, Howes does not discuss this finding in any great detail, focusing instead on the material motivations (wages, benefits) that draw aides into caregiving. Howes is not alone in her singular focus on the economic rewards and constraints of paid care work. In general, those interested in aggregate trends in the home care workforce acknowledge the subjective motivations of workers but do not comprehensively measure or analyze them.

While it is significant that researchers have established the centrality of wages and benefits to worker recruitment and retention, I suggest it is also important to study the nonmaterial factors that matter to nursing aides. In his book *Dignity at Work*, Randy Hodson (2001) implores sociologists to examine how workers craft meaning and self-purpose on the job—in a word, dignity—often in the context of significant physical and emotional constraint. He identifies four behavioral domains used by workers to safeguard dignity at work, two of which are particularly germane to this discussion: the pursuit of meaning and social relations at work (17). Hodson argues that workers seek to find meaning and purpose in their work "outside the institutionally scripted flow of organizational activity"

(18). That is, workers impart their own values, meaning systems, interpretations, and actions into work as a way of claiming ownership and control over their labor. Similarly, workers rely on social relationships—with co-workers, customers, or clients—to derive meaning out of work that might otherwise alienate or deny dignity.

Home care aides interviewed for this book speak to the significance of meaning making and social ties at work. Even in the context of low occupational prestige and poor wages, home care aides assign meaning to their physical and emotional labor so as to remind themselves, and others, of the social value of their work. Andrew, for example, is motivated by both wages and a commitment to serving his client. Andrew concedes that the low wages and physical strain of the job are serious constraints to his overall job satisfaction, but he also believes that his work positively impacts the lives of his clients and, by extension, the broader public. He tells me:

> Where would Rusty be right now if I wasn't here? He would be in a facility. His mother, she's sixty-four years old. She just remarried and she openly came here and said, "I don't want to deal with him." She has a life of her own. So where would he be? He'd be up in a facility where the state would have to be paying, wow, how much money? About five thousand dollars a month just to care for him. It's cheaper for the state to pay me.

Aides in this study construct meaning at work in three primary ways: by describing their care as a natural ability or gift, by framing their care as a service to others, and by drawing clear social boundaries between themselves and "uncaring" others. Through this "vocabulary of motive" (Mills 1940) aides affirm their social utility while also constructing a sense of self on the job. This situated identity is what I mean by the term *the caring self*. Like all situated identities (Mills 1940; Holstein and Gubrium 2000), the caring self is formed in relation to aides' specific social location and conditioned by the environment in which they work, that is, the private homes of clients. In this work-home space, aides find a great deal of autonomy to define and provide care "on their own terms" with little interference from superiors or family. In addition, aides often form fictive kinship ties with clients, further cementing the informal nature of the work relationship. These two factors—autonomy at work and fictive kinship—are important conditions for the caring self. An important third factor that shapes the caring self is social location. While aides have their occupation in common, there are important variations in the caring self that emerge by race and ethnicity. The remainder of this chapter explores in detail the different dimensions of the caring self, paying particular attention to the way in which worker accounts are shaped by the informal context of care.

I suggest it is important to study aides' subjective accounts of work and self for two reasons. First, if sociologists are to understand how inequalities of labor sustain over time, we must engage the question of how social actors on the ground make sense of their structurally disadvantaged positions. To do so allows us to understand how workers—in this case low-wage health care aides—adapt to or challenge the limits of opportunity. Second, if policymakers aim to create and sustain a quality workforce in long-term care, it is first useful to understand what *material* and *nonmaterial* rewards foster recruitment and retention. Although aides speak on occasion about issues of burnout and job satisfaction, they are far more animated about their emotional bonds to clients. If, as many scholars have postulated, burnout is tied to the emotional overextension of workers (Erickson 1995; Wharton 1999), an important first step in reducing the rate of burnout and turnover is to understand the nature of aides' emotional commitments to clients. Only then can scholars and policymakers tease out which dimensions of the caregiver-client interaction deplete aides' physical or emotional resources and which ones foster job satisfaction, a positive sense of self, and dignity.

Autonomy at Work

One of the key contextual factors of the caring self is the degree of autonomy home care aides have on the job, especially relative to their counterparts working in institutional care. Although the job of home care worker offers relatively low pay and little vertical mobility, workers have a great deal of freedom to direct their work and control the degree of emotional energy they put into their care. The home care agencies discussed here generally take a "hands-off" approach to the management of aides, requiring only that aides fill out a checklist of completed tasks for each visit (IHSS does not require even this). In the for-profit company It's For You, located in Central City, California, licensed vocational nurses

(LVNs) do make unannounced house calls to ensure that clients are well cared for and that aides are on-site. I learned from both the nurses and home care aides that these "check-ins" rarely lead to the dismissal of an aide. Reported incidents are rare, at least according to the supervisors and managers of the agencies under study, and most of the time caregivers and clients are left alone to negotiate work tasks on a day-to-day basis. Home care workers resemble temporary workers in this regard: in both cases the work is highly decentralized, autonomous, and relies on self-monitoring rather than direct managerial supervision (V. Smith 1998; Smith and Neuwirth 2008).

IHSS, administered by the county, is run on a consumer-driven model and encourages the client to take responsibility for the hiring, training, and firing of an aide. As a consequence, aides have an employer of record (the county) and an on-site employer who must direct care (the elderly or disabled client). In this case, as well as in the private agencies, aides are at a remove from the employer who pays their wage. Therefore it is not uncommon for elderly or disabled clients to be completely unaware of rates of pay and type of benefits aides receive in exchange for their labor. Depending on the situation, clients and their families might "manage" aides and assume responsibility for their dismissal or training, though clients are often too physically or mentally weak, or lack the management skills, to direct their own care in this way.

Not surprisingly, medical liability in this context is muddy at best. Private agencies like It's For You screen their aides carefully and periodically monitor their work through "drop-ins" carried out by LVNs or RNs. IHSS is a much larger organization to administer and control, not to mention the fact that the program must provide care to seniors and disabled individuals too poor to pay for it. Counties serve as employers of record for home care workers but assume no liability if a client is abused or hurt as a result of caregiver negligence. The "hands-off" approach of IHSS is partially a result of the structural constraints placed on the state agency to provide care for an increasing number of people at minimal cost to the state and taxpayer. For this reason, issues of liability take a backseat to the problem of simply finding enough caregivers to meet the needs of an ever-expanding elderly population. As one administrator commented during an informal interview, home care at the county level is an "accident waiting to happen" due to the unregulated nature of care and the short supply of county social workers and public health nurses available to monitor cases.

Although there are potential problems associated with the lack of supervision aides receive—such as elder abuse, substandard care, or exploitation of aides—autonomy is a crucial factor in aides' job satisfaction and identity construction. Aides experience two types of autonomy: functional autonomy and relational autonomy. Both work to give aides a sense of control over their labor, especially relative to prior work experiences in the service sector, and lay the foundation for the construction of the caring self at work.

Functional Autonomy

In *Dignity and Work*, Randy Hodson (2001) reviews the ethnographic literature on autonomy in the workplace and concludes that workers experience autonomy in patterned ways, dependent on the context of work. In professional and craft settings, workers experience high autonomy, creativity, and job satisfaction relative to workers in bureaucratic settings or those in environments managed by supervisory fiat. Craft workers, for example, possess a "functional autonomy," or the "necessary skills to ensure that production proceeds correctly and efficiently" (Hodson 2001, 141). Professionals assert autonomy based more on an expert body of knowledge that allows them to define the terms of work without management intervention. As a caveat to these observations, Hodson adds that women are more likely to work in environments with low levels of autonomy and creativity, and this significantly compromises their dignity in the workplace (167).

Nursing aides working in institutions have little direct or functional autonomy over their work, since nurse managers generally control and monitor their labor (Diamond 1992; Foner 1994; Lopez 2006). Home care aides, in contrast, have a high degree of autonomy with respect to their freedom from direct supervision and their control over the timing, pace, and scope of work. With respect to latitude to make decisions and assert occupational discretion, aides formally have low degrees of autonomy, but they are able to exercise judgment and discretion when circumstance permits or demands, such as during a medical emergency.

Aides seek out and welcome the direct control they have over work tasks, schedules, and even their on-the-job attire. Many aides describe autonomy as a feeling of "being your own boss" or the freedom to establish work routines without supervision. In the context of both IHSS and the two for-profit agencies, all aides—in some way or another—place high priority on having control over the direction of care. Mark, an Asian American man in his forties, works for IHSS and is also employed by several clients privately. He explains autonomy in this way:

> Yes, you can almost say I am my own boss. Yes, I have someone over me. I mean, everyone has someone over them sooner or later. But you have the flexibility to run your own schedule, set your own times to a certain degree, and pray, hope that, if you are like me, you don't overbook and cross over somebody else's schedule.

Virginia identifies autonomy as one of the key reasons she stays in the job but acknowledges that freedom over work rules and routines is not for everyone. She describes why autonomy is important to her:

> I guess the freedom of the job, you know, you call your own shots, you don't have anyone breathing down your neck. But there are people that maybe can't work without somebody telling them the rules, reminding them to be on time, and that kind of thing. Some people need to have a more structured area to work in. For me, I've always been honest. You know, I know what my job is supposed to be and I go and do it. And I like that freedom.

Maggie has something similar to say about freedom on the job. She has worked in nursing homes and in home care and prefers the latter, with a strong preference for private-pay clients. She tells me, "I'd rather do it on my own because you're not so stressed out. You have a little more leeway, more freedom. You don't have people down your neck." Mary also appreciates the freedom she has to make decisions while on the job. Although her client, Rose, provides some input, Mary is generally in control of the pace and scope of her work:

> I'm just kind of on my own and I decide the kind of day, what I'm going to do, which is kind of nice. If I don't do what Rose wants, she'll ask me and I'll do it. But it's kind of like I have my own routine when I go in. It's almost like being in my own house.

Shelly likes the fact that she can wear what she would like to work, which in turn allows her to express her "true self" while she provides care to others:

> There are not so many rules and regulations [in home care]. I'm allowed to wear tank tops. I'm allowed to wear piercings. And everybody loves me just same. I don't have to pretend I'm somebody I'm not. I still wear scrubs, you know, and I still dress professionally, but I'm not going to be somebody I'm not to please somebody else.

Jennifer is an aide who "lives in" with her client, an elderly woman in her eighties, and is paid to provide around-the-clock care. Although Jennifer's life revolves around care for her elderly client, Diane, the job affords Jennifer a great deal of flexibility, allowing her to take continuing-education classes at night:

> They [the agency and family] are very flexible. As long as I take care of her, I have my evenings free, and I have quite a long period in the evening that I can go to get education [training] like that, and as long as I get back by, you know, a reasonable time, nine, ten o'clock at night, it's fine.

Jennifer's fondness for her current job makes even further sense when placed in the context of her broader work history. She tells of how her former job as an assistant to a workaholic insurance adjuster made her chronically ill. The long hours, stress, and what she calls "mind games" led, she says, to an autoimmune disease and chronic fatigue. She explains:

> I was just too stressed, and the pressure. And you get in that rat race and you just can't get out of it, and there is just no end to people demanding things from you, and you have to put up with so much junk from people, so much crap. That's the only way I know how to explain it; just shit piles on and piles on you, and you have to try and make everybody happy, and you can't make anybody happy because they're all mad.

Jennifer "found" caregiving when she needed a job after leaving the insurance business and a friend offered to pay her minimum wage to look after her father, who had just suffered a heart attack. Jennifer found the work to be manageable and "rewarding," and she eventually sought out full-time employment with IHSS.

As such testimonies illustrate, aides benefit from autonomy in a direct sense: they are given a certain degree of freedom to set the terms of their employment and to independently schedule work tasks. These realities appear positively linked to aides' overall job satisfaction. Aides also describe a less favorable autonomy by default that stems from the simple fact that no one else is around to take care of client needs. As we learned in chapter 2, home care aides are often the only ones present when a medical situation arises, and so are left with the responsibility of providing hands-on care to clients. While agencies are careful to formally remind aides that providing certain services, like changing catheters, injecting insulin, and administering first aid, is forbidden, in practice agencies take a "don't ask, don't tell" approach to monitoring aides. The aides I spoke with and observed are aware that the inattentiveness of agencies gives them autonomy to provide the kind of care normally off-limits to health care workers of their skill level, but many worry that such autonomy might result in harm to a client, job loss, or reprimand by agencies. In short, aides' direct autonomy over work tasks is somewhat of a mixed blessing, resulting in both job satisfaction and workplace anxiety.

Interviews with visiting nurses working for IHSS confirm that aides are in effect, and only by default, given the autonomy to provide minor medical care to clients simply because there is no one else to do it. Most nurses express frustration that their own scope of work is restricted because, as field nurses, they do not work directly under a doctor's order. Aides, of course, do not work under a doctor's order either, but their relative invisibility in the medical hierarchy seems to paradoxically give them greater autonomy to tend to clients' bodies in ways that even nurses cannot. Of the nine nurses interviewed, all expressed deep concerns that this autonomy by default leads to the neglect and abuse of clients, although only one nurse could recall a specific instance. Aides are aware that nurses and other medical professionals see them in this way but justify their autonomy as a necessary part of the care of clients, whose minor medical needs otherwise go untreated. What appears unrecognized by all parties is that home care workers now absorb a great deal of responsibility and risk by taking on work that extends beyond the limits of their training. While this autonomy gives aides a degree of job satisfaction, there is also considerable risk involved for both clients and caregivers.

Relational Autonomy

Not unlike craft or professional workers, home care aides gain dignity and job satisfaction through independent control over work practices (Hodson 2001). In addition to this functional autonomy, aides also cultivate *relational autonomy* (Parks 2003), which allows them to invest emotionally in their clients, on their own terms. Jobs like teaching, nursing, domestic work, and home care—in which women are disproportionately represented—all contain components of autonomy as well as "relationality" (Chodorow 1978) that converge to produce or limit workplace dignity. Jennifer Parks (2003) names women's autonomy in the context of care work "relational autonomy," a concept I borrow here in the discussion of home care. For aides, relational autonomy is not simply the ability to act independently of others, but rather the ability to *act for others* without undue constraint.

Acting for others is obviously central to the work of home care aides, but it is the emotional (rather than physical) acts that workers see as most important. Specifically, aides purposefully cultivate companionship with their clients, engaging in a set of relational practices to ensure that a connection is made and sustained. Caregivers appreciate that home care allows them to build relationships with clients over time and in a genuine way. Tammy, for instance, spends time "puttering" around her elderly client's home, talking about the woman's childhood and family dramas of the moment. Realizing that others may not see this as work, Tammy insists that a great deal of energy goes into listening and relating to her client, a part of the job she relishes. "I really could write her story," she says. "And that's a wonderful thing. I mean, I love the stories."

Other aides share Tammy's sentiments in their own work situations. Mary says she struggled to find meaningful work after experiencing a divorce in her late fifties that left her broke, in debt, and with no income. After trying a number of different jobs, Mary settled on home care in large part because of the relational aspects of the work, specifically the talking and listening required of aides:

I think it's really important. It really is, because you've got to nurture these people.... They don't have a lot, they don't have many people coming into their lives to build them up and nurture them.... You know, they just, they need that. Or if they want us to talk about their family issues and stuff, it's someone to talk to about it.... It's companionship.

Cultivating companionship is arguably the most crucial part of the home care aide's job and it is what sets her apart from other institution-based careworkers who are prohibited, or in some cases discouraged, from forming strong bonds with patients (Diamond 1992; Foner 1994). After working months or years in a nursing home or other facility, many aides sever ties with institutions and actively search for a job that allows for greater relational autonomy. Aides cite poor working conditions and neglect of patients as the central reasons for leaving institutional care. They recount emotional stories of working eight- or ten-hour shifts without a break and feeling as though, no matter how hard they tried, clients did not receive the proper care. Most describe a "tipping point," after which they could no longer stomach institutional work. For many aides, home care became the place where they could exercise both functional and relational autonomy. This reality becomes clear when aides describe in detail the constraints on autonomy experienced in nursing homes.

José, who has a CNA license, worked for years in institutional care and took issue with the way that both clients and workers were treated. He found the "speedup" of work particularly difficult to manage:

A lot of places, the workers don't have the time, there's not enough time in the day to do it. Me, I didn't have much time either because I hardly got to lunch. I had maybe a fifteen-minute break in my whole shift because I had to make sure these people were right. Taking into account that they are going to give low man on the totem pole all the patients that no one else wants. It's hard for you to dedicate enough time for each one of the residents.

Mary is another aide who moved from an institutional setting to home-based care. She took her first paid caregiving job in an assisted living facility, but determined quickly that she could not handle the pace of work. Routinely working the second shift, Mary found herself in charge of fifteen or more patients a night without any breaks or support from other staff. She recalls "plopping" residents in front of the TV in the activity room simply so she could complete her tasks of bathing and changing each person under her charge. Mary left the job when the aide-to-patient ratio began to climb. Her daughter still works at the facility, where the ratio on the second shift is now one aide for every thirty patients. Viewing this ratio as "ridiculous," Mary vows to never work another day in a facility. At sixty-seven, she says she will leave this type of caregiving to younger aides who can handle the physical and mental toil of the job.

Virginia believes, like Mary, that she is physically and emotionally unfit for work in a nursing home. She recalls one of her first shifts in an assisted living facility where she was left to care for twelve patients on her own. Describing the situation as "like the Keystone Kops, no, Three Stooges," Virginia had trouble keeping up with the pace of the work while also ensuring that the residents were properly cared for. With a touch of self-deprecation in her voice, Virginia told of her frustrated efforts to change an elderly woman with atrophied muscles into a nightgown. Although she had encountered similar situations in home care, Virginia felt acute pressure to move quickly and get to the next resident. In her mind, the pace of work prevented her from making connections with the elderly women and men under her care:

> I move a little slower, and I like to give. I told them [at the facility], I said, "You don't want me back. I know you don't want me back." I mean, my heart was in it, but I just couldn't do the speed, to get everybody ready.... I'm good at what I do. And I can move and groove. I can get four or five a day [in home care] and get them done and keep going. But I just couldn't do *that*.

When I ask Virginia if she thinks that aides who work in nursing homes are somehow less connected to their work or their patients, she makes clear that while there are always "bad ones," the vast majority of aides working in nursing homes are conscientious people constrained by a poor work environment:

> It seems like there's good people out there...there are. You always hear about the bad ones. But, you know, some of these aides are so devoted to their patients, and really care about them and get attached to them. And I felt that way about the ones I did in home care. But it's horrible what happens with [aides]. And the sad part is [the nursing homes] don't want to pay. With what they're charging these people to be in those homes, and what

they pay an aide or a nurse to be in there, I think it's horrible. It is. It's ridiculous. You got them in there, you're getting that kind of money, where's that money going?

Virginia acknowledges that there are aides who aren't "nice," but she sees this as more a problem of life circumstances and work conditions rather than a personal failing. She suggests that "maybe they just become not-such-a-nice person because [the nursing homes] burn her out. She can't feed her family, you know. I take my hat off. I do." Virginia will remain in home care until she retires, leaving the facility work to younger women who, she says, can handle the pace and emotional detachment.

Like Virginia, Shelly finds it nearly impossible to provide high-quality care to clients without "cutting corners," something she is unwilling to do. She describes how conditions at nursing homes undermine her own ethic of care and beliefs about the humanity of patients:

> Each shift, everybody had a side, and you had at least two to four showers, as well as getting people up and changing them, getting them dressed for the day, depending on what shift. Every two hours [the residents] are changed and pottied, unless, of course, they say they have to go sooner or they were incontinent. But not everybody follows those rules. You know, there are corners that you have to cut when working there. But I don't believe that people should be left messy and, you know, in their own waste.... These are people.

Later in our conversation, I ask Shelly why she remains in home care even though the pay is better at assisted living facilities. She replies that home care "is cool. It is what you make of it." She adds, "I could be really depressed that I don't make any money. But that's not why I'm in it. I could go to the hospital and make twice what I'm making now. But I don't. That's not the kind of job that I want."

Shelly's comment that home care "is what you make of it" is a frequently heard aphorism among aides, but in the context of her broader comments also indicates that Shelly finds a greater degree of relational autonomy in home care, where she is relatively free to invest in the well-being of clients. Like Shelly, most aides are aware that they could make more money in assisted living facilities or nursing homes, but they still choose home care where they can provide care on their own terms. Shelly explains that compared to nursing or working as an aide in an institution, "you actually do more work with patients by doing [home care]. I have it way better. It's awesome."

Camilla, a thirty-nine-year-old African American aide, expresses similar sentiments about why she chooses home care over institutional care:

> To me [a nursing home is] too busy. It's not enough time for the client. You know what I mean? You have no personal time with them. You are going to give them a bath real quick, check their temperature, blood pressure, and you're out of there. What about "How do you feel today?" or "Did you sleep well? Did you have any dreams?" "Is there anything bothering you?" You know, rub their head and take time to do all that. The important stuff. And that's what I do.

Camilla finds that home care gives her the relational autonomy to provide for the physical and mental needs of her client. Maggie feels similarly about the connections she is able to make with clients in home care. In her assessment, "You get to be more personal [in home care]. You get to be close, real close to the people and family. Institutional is altogether different. You can't have that little closeness like you do with somebody in their own home." Like Camilla and Maggie, aides fleeing work in long-term care facilities see home-based work as a way to privilege their own ethic of care, free of bureaucratic constraint.

Paid caregivers welcome the relational autonomy characteristic of home care precisely because they are free to care according to their own standards. Patty is an aide who takes care of Ed, an elderly man who lives alone in Middletown. Each day Patty bathes, cleans, and feeds Ed, working approximately four hours per day for him. On the weekends, Patty finds herself worrying about Ed's well-being, since he generally relies on his neighbors for help when she is "off duty." Last spring, Patty woke up on a Saturday morning and convinced her husband to drive with her over to Ed's house, just to check on him briefly. Patty and her husband found Ed in his garden, enjoying the warm weather but lamenting the state of his yard. Before long, Patty and her husband had outlined landscaping plans with Ed, which then turned into a "quick trip" to a home and garden store, followed by a long afternoon of planting flowers and a few shrubs on Ed's property. Patty feels good for helping Ed, even without compensation, but simultaneously worries that she is breaking the rules of the agency (which she is).

Most aides are aware that agencies prohibit them from caring for clients in off-hours, but like Patty, a number of them cite their "right to care" as a way of dismissing agency rules and regulations. Tammy, also from Middletown, currently has a client who is temporarily living in a skilled nursing facility after a recent surgery. The client will eventually return home and Tammy will resume care for her at that point. In the interim, Tammy accepts regular phone calls from the client, who is feeling lonely. About this breech in the rules, Tammy says, "She calls me several times a week from the nursing home, which is not allowed. But I allow it so we can stay in touch. [Supervisors at the agency] really discourage it. We're not supposed to give out our phones, but that's my business. What I do with my phone is my business."

As these accounts demonstrate, autonomy in a setting of interdependency looks very different from what we might identify as autonomy in other professions. Home care aides experience creativity and self-determination through relational autonomy (Parks 2003) where decisions are always made in the context of another person's needs. This leads to situations where aides experience the greatest creativity and self-determination on the job precisely in those moments when they extend to meet needs of a dependent person. Findings are consistent with earlier work on nursing home aides that suggest some segment of workers will always seek out ways to promote high standards, even in the face of structural pressures to prioritize profit over care (Diamond 1992).

For some of the aides interviewed, relational autonomy is more about the ability to control and anticipate emotionality on the job. Just as aides in home care have greater latitude to extend care to clients, they are also more likely than their institutional counterparts to foresee and prepare for emotionally charged situations. Patty, an aide in Ohio, dislikes nursing homes because she gets "so emotionally attached to clients" and fears that she would have to routinely deal with unanticipated death. While she concedes that the passing of clients is a part of home care as well, she believes that she will know when her client is approaching death and be able to prepare herself emotionally. Patty also feels that shifts and work tasks change so regularly at nursing homes that she would be emotionally hurt when relationships necessarily changed or were severed without her input. In home care, Patty is able to acquaint herself with clients over time and without any real fear of sudden change to the relationships. She adds that she would be very "angry" if her employer, an agency in Middletown, took her away from her clients without warning. For Patty, working in home care ensures that when she invests emotionally in clients, she can witness the rewards of this investment over time without intervention from a third party.

Both direct and relational autonomy contribute to job satisfaction and workplace dignity for home care aides. In particular, relational autonomy allows aides to provide care on their own terms and develop sustained emotional connections to clients. In a more general sense, these accounts show us that relational autonomy is a way in which aides maneuver for greater job satisfaction within the lower tier of the service sector. There is a fine line, however, between aides' autonomy and the exploitation of their impulse to care. Aides are given latitude to care as they see fit, at least relative to aides working in institutions, but sometimes this means that their surplus labor goes unnoticed or uncompensated. Dropping by a client's house on the weekend or accepting after-hour phone calls can be simultaneously interpreted as expressions of workplace autonomy or as exploitative work conditions. This tension between autonomy and exploitation is very real in home care, precisely because it is an example of "marketized private life"(Hochschild 2003) in which the blurring of boundaries between home and work lead to confused social norms, work obligations, and feeling rules. This confused home/work arrangement potentially benefits aides, giving them greater autonomy over care, but it can also contribute to the inequality of an already disenfranchised class of worker.

Fictive Kinship

Aides routinely use terms like "grandma," "mother," and "sister" to describe their relationships with clients. Beyond these descriptive labels, however, aides also act in ways reminiscent of kin when in client homes. These "fictive kin" ties (Karner 1998; Lan 2002; Stack 1974) are sources of pride and dignity for aides who see themselves as "filling in" for absent family members. Additionally, fictive kinship is an important contextual factor in the construction of the caring self, since family ties with clients help cement the notion that aides are naturally inclined to provide care, just as daughters, mothers, or grandmothers might be.

When clients live alone and have few others to rely on, aides remark that friend or family bonds form quickly and naturally. As Mary puts it:

"To me, I can't help but build a relationship with them because I care about them. Like as a friend." Similarly, Patty likens one of the clients to her now-deceased grandfather, commenting, "He [the client] is kind of like the grandparent. I don't have my grandparent anymore, so he's kind of like...you know, an old, cute guy."

Tammy cared for her neighbor Sue, a middle-aged woman with multiple sclerosis, for nearly five years. Sue had never married, had no children, and was living far from her own elderly parents. Tammy became Sue's around-the-clock caregiver, despite the fact that their prior relationship consisted of a few "over the fence" conversations. Ultimately, the two formed a close bond that Tammy compared to a sibling relationship, replete with all the tensions and interpersonal dynamics customary between sisters:

> She really did depend on that daily contact with me. Several of her friends kept in touch by phone, and that helped a lot. But I found that I actually had to play the big sister a lot of times, and get bossy, and tell her what to do. You know, "You have to take your meds. You have to eat." She would go days without eating....It was much like a sibling relationship in that she would take so much motivation from me, and then shut me down. "That's enough!" Which I loved; I really enjoyed that part.

Tammy certainly felt a great deal of emotional stress as a result of her bond with Sue, but she also believes there are considerable psychosocial benefits that come from knowing a client so intimately:

> I don't think many people have an opportunity to know someone that deeply. I really honestly think there is nothing that we didn't talk about. We just—there are no holds barred. And to get to know somebody at that level....I don't even know my husband or my children at that level. So that's the benefit. And I wouldn't give that up for anything.

Andrew, the aide profiled at the beginning of the chapter, recalls the fictive bonds formed with several of his elderly male clients. Describing the relationships, Andrew struggles to find a way to capture the nature of the connection:

> We came to where we just clash and argue and have disputes, and that's going to happen, you know, and then we become friends again and make

up. Every client I have ever had, every one, we've had clashes like that, arguments, disputes. Bernie and I were so close, you know? If I needed money or anything, he'd go, "What you need?" and let me have a thousand and I'd pay it back. Need fifteen hundred dollars or whatever? He was real smart, you know? Breaking up with him was like, you know, breaking up from your wife or something. You have established that kind of relationship, you know, when you're kind of breaking away from somebody. Like I had one person I'd go over there day and night, that was the last person I'd see at night. I'd put them in bed, and you're married, you know. It's not like being gay, it's a different type of—it's like you're family or something.

Although the idea of fictive kinship rests in part on the idea that aides are filling a gap left by absent family, it is also usually the case that immediate and extended families help reinforce the notion that aides are "one of the family." Dot, for example, cared for a disabled woman in her fifties and found that the client's husband and daughter both welcomed, even expected, Dot to act as family. She explains:

Even though you were taking care of her, she [the client] really made you feel part of the family. She was very, very social. And then of course her husband! I made her a special lunch every day, and he'd actually go out and buy me, you know, meals that I wanted for lunch. It was just like part of family. Even her daughter, when she was in college, she was home for the summer and still made you feel like you're just part of the family. They were just very nice people. And Margaret, she was just a very elegant lady.

When I suggest that such a relationship with a client and her family might be exceptional, Dot counters with several other examples from her nearly thirty-year career as an aide. She explains that "in home care...some clients you're with five or six years, and it gets to be more than just—it gets to be really personal after that." Even when clients take a turn for the worse and end up in the hospital, Dot does not see this as the end of the caregiver-client relationship. At one point during the study, an elderly client of hers ended up very ill and needed care beyond Dot's expertise. Even so, Dot saw the client regularly, and offered me the following explanation: "I still went to see her at the nursing home. It was just like my little family."

Camilla, who we met earlier in this chapter, formed a close relationship with one of her elderly clients and his family. After working for the family, through an agency, for nearly a year, Camilla became a central part of the end-of-life care for her client, even sharing in his last few moments of life. In her retelling of events, it is clear that Camilla is moved by the degree to which the family included her in the very private process of ushering a loved one through the dying process:

> They wanted me to be there all the time. And then the daughter says, "Please, you can just spend the night; spend the night." They were so comfortable with me there; it was so amazing to me. It didn't matter to me. "Whatever you want. You can call me in the middle of the night. You want me to come back, I will. It doesn't matter," you know? Until he died. And I was right there with them, the whole family.

Maggie spoke at length about her days working as an aide in Kentucky, before she moved to Ohio nearly ten years ago. She has fond memories of working with clients who treated her as family and, as she points out, "not as an employee":

> I got attached to a blind lady that I took care of in Kentucky. Her family just treated me like family. Then I had a lady that was one hundred years old, very sharp. Everyday she made notes: who was coming in her house, who was leaving, what was going on. Her family treated me just like family. I wasn't treated like an employee. They'd go away, and then they'd bring me back gifts and everything. And then I had a retired schoolteacher I took care of. I was treated like family through everybody that I knew in Kentucky. I mean, it was just wonderful. I was not treated like an employee at all. I was just part of the family.

Maggie is less enthusiastic about the last decade of her caregiving career in Ohio. Since the move north, Maggie feels more like an employee than a family member to her clients. She attributes this difference to the agencies with whom she contracted in Ohio. In Kentucky, Maggie secured paid care work informally, by word of mouth, and generally received better pay. On moving to Ohio, Maggie experienced a series of workplace injuries that left her with agonizing back pain, unable to work for weeklong stretches at a time. As a result, Maggie's financial situation has been precarious in recent years, a situation exacerbated by the circumstances of her oldest son, who relies on her to help pay for his own medical bills. Maggie recently moved into an apartment complex for low-income seniors and has already begun informally looking for clients there. She hopes to find elders in the complex who need help with activities of daily living and are without family to assist.

Maggie's case is interesting because it raises the question of whether aides form fictive kinship bonds with clients in part because they lack familial networks and support of their own. In other words, is fictive kinship instigated and sustained—perhaps even imagined—by aides who themselves need emotional support? Although not all aides readily elaborated on their family lives and histories, some patterns are discernible. Aides over the age of sixty, for example, talk about being able to relate to the health and emotional needs of their clients, a factor that blurs distinctions between clients and caregivers. Mary, for example, feels like she has a "reciprocal" relationship with Darla, a client ten years her senior who she views as a "close friend." They swap stories about their respective "family problems"(both are divorced) and their various aches and pains. Mary sometimes worries that their relationship is too much like a friendship or sibling relationship and that she "probably shares too much." Although the agency prohibits aides from sharing personal stories with clients, Mary feels such a rule is impractical: "When you kind of build up that friendship level, it's hard not to share things." Although many of the younger aides also report strong fictive family bonds with clients, they tend not to see the relationship as reciprocal. Instead, younger aides view themselves as filling a care gap left by absent family or, alternatively, as playing a crucial role in a family's efforts to provide quality care to a loved one.

Even with these subtle differences between younger and older caregivers, the general finding remains that, irrespective of age and social background, aides use the language of family to describe the depth of their caring commitments. Fictive kinship provides an important foundation for the caring self because the identity is constructed around aides' beliefs that care is a *service to others* they are uniquely ordained to carry out. The common belief that caregiving is a service to "family" also helps sustain aides' narratives of care as a natural or innate gift, an extension of their roles as parents, spouses, siblings, and children. In short, fictive kinship expands the altruistic and service dimensions of the caring

self in ways that a more formal employer-employee relationship likely
would not.

Constructing the Caring Self

The importance aides give to both relational autonomy and fictive family
ties when they talk about their work points to a larger sociological reality:
workplaces are important sites of identity construction. Just as our "situated selves" (Mills 1940) are crafted at school, in church, and in the family,
identities are equally, if not more, influenced by the context of work. Sociologists use many terms to theorize and explain the social nature of identity
construction. I borrow Snow and Anderson's term "identity work" to refer
to the general process by which home care aides "create, present, and sustain
personal identities" (Snow and Anderson 1987, 1348). Central to identity
work is "identity talk," or the verbal construction and assertion of identity.
Similar to Mills's (1940) vocabularies of motive, identity talk reflects how
low-status social actors narrate a sense of self to others, in the hope of preserving a sense of self-worth and dignity (Snow and Anderson 1987).

Home care workers engage in identity work (broadly) and identity talk
(specifically) with the particular aim of reinforcing the *caring self*.[1] The caring self is a situated identity that aides actively construct on the job as a way
of communicating to themselves and others that their work is altruistically
motivated and of high quality. Aides achieve the caring self through three
types of identity talk: professing their care as natural or innate, emphasizing service to others, and drawing boundaries between themselves and
"uncaring others."

Caring as Natural Ability, Gift, or Calling

An important part of constructing the caring self is making clear to one-
self and others that proclivities to caregiving are deep-seated components
of personality or natural traits present from birth. Most of the women, and
some of the men, who end up in home care have caring trajectories that
involve years of informal care of friends and family, realities that limit as
much as they foster occupational opportunity. Even so, aides generally view
their caring trajectory as clear reflection of innate talents for caregiving.

As such, working in home care is narrated as an outgrowth of firmly held convictions and natural talents, rather than an indication of constrained choices in a service economy.

Dot, from Middletown, believes that she has possessed a set of relational skills from childhood that make her well suited to caregiving, such as her ability to talk and listen to older people:

> To me, I find it very fascinating. And I love talking to people; I'm a people person. I always have been. But I have my times too. I like my privacy, just like everybody else. But I don't know.... I've always been attracted to older people. People seem to come to me; I mean they just talk. And I'm a great listener.

Maggie recalls that she too has a long-standing affinity for older people:

> Well, I've always cared about the older people, even when I was young. I just found them very interesting. They tell stories about their lives and the things that they've done, and it was just very interesting to me. I was always closer to older people for some reason.

And Camilla believes that her ability to relate to older people is "a gift" possessed only by a select few:

> It's easy for me. I believe that it's a gift. It can be learned, but everybody don't have the patience for it. And they don't have the right attitude for it. You have to understand where they [the elderly] are coming from.

With extended careers in paid care work, Dot, Maggie, and Camilla are certain of their caregiving skills and their natural affinities for elder care. Aides newer to the work rely on others to help reinforce the idea that they are "born to care." Tammy, after caring for her neighbor Sue for five years and then losing her to multiple sclerosis, felt aimless and unsure of how to occupy her time in the year after Sue's death. Although Tammy spent much of her adult life caring for others without pay—her children, her own parents—it was through interaction with close friends that her view of herself as a natural caregiver was reinforced:

> Another friend of mine made a comment to me one day. I was apparently being a little too motherly and sisterly with my friend Kathleen, and she

said, "You know, I really think you need...somebody to take care of." And it just made perfect sense to me. And I have always been that way, even as a child I was a nurturer..., you know, a cat rescuer, and took care of things. It made sense, and I decided to try it [working for an agency]. I got back into it, and I just loved it. It was the right thing to do.

Kristen has nursed seven close family members through terminal illness and death. The last fifteen years of her life have been punctuated by obligations to family that include caring for her husband after triple bypass surgery, moving in with her parents to help them manage cancer and Alzheimer's, providing around-the-clock care to her husband's sister who died of cancer, and commuting a considerable distance to take care of a niece with a malignant brain tumor. In short, Kristen became the "one to call" in her family if anyone fell ill. A devout Christian and proud political conservative, Kristen believes she possesses a gift for compassion that disposes her to the task of formal and informal caregiving. In her view, women are both responsible for care and the best suited to carry out the work.

Kristen's conviction that women are naturally disposed to care for others is, of course, grounded in wider social beliefs about women's obligation to care for children and dependent elders (Aronson 1992; Gordon, Benner, and Noddings 1996). While many of the aides question the fairness of pay or the rules and regulations of agencies, not a single aide spoke critically about gender norms that reinforce women's roles as caregivers. Rather, aides themselves invoke gendered beliefs about caring to justify and explain their own caring careers, both formal and informal. Sally, an African American aide working in Central City, for example, doesn't even use the word "caregiver" when describing her work. She feels that assigning herself such a title sullies the essential quality of her caregiving role: "Oh, no, I don't tell people I'm a caregiver, even though I receive a check for caregiving and did it for many years. But to give myself a title? No. Females *are* caregivers."

For a subset of the caregivers, it is clear that religion reinforces a "natural" division of labor when it comes to caregiving. Jennifer, who recently became a born-again Christian, says that few are surprised about her caregiving path because she has always had a "maternal instinct." When asked to elaborate, she responds:

I'm very much a caregiver, this is my nature, and I knew there had to be a situation out there for me, it was just a matter of finding it....Everything is planned for you from the time you are born until the time you die, and you have things that you have to go through.... I know that God has given me a path and he's shown me the way.

Jennifer's religious conviction confirms, and extends, Cinzia Solari's (2006) observation that home care workers vary in their orientations to care based on religion and cultural tradition: Jewish caregivers emphasize "professionalism," while Christians call themselves "saints." While Solari's sample is limited to Russian immigrants only, I suggest that religious conviction helps reinforce for some aides that caregiving is natural for women. By investing in and sustaining a religious sensibility in their care work, aides construct care as "women's work" and themselves as pious servants. Such religious justification for women's paid labor is not unique to home care. As Bethany Moreton (2009) shows in her book about Walmart, Christian notions of family and service are present among store clerks, who view their interactive labor with customers as an act of devotion.

Home care aides construct a sense of self on the job—a caring self—in part by narrating care work as a natural or innate component of their personalities. Calling on traditional gender norms, and to a lesser extent on religious conviction, home care workers make it known to themselves and others that their care work is an expression of a true self. In so doing, aides contribute to the belief that caring for others is a product of deep-seated personality traits or natural impulses to care. This subjective viewpoint of caregivers exists awkwardly alongside the structural reality of aides' lives and job opportunities. Home care aides follow "career lines" (Spenner, Otto, and Call 1982) that position them in low-wage jobs with limited opportunity for mobility. These career lines or trajectories begin with a history of providing informal care to family or friends without pay and then ultimately translate, at various stages in the life course, to poorly compensated care work in the formal economy. While each aide constructs and justifies her own employment biography in terms that make sense to her and allow for positive identity construction at work, these biographies also point to a series of "constrained choices" over the life course (Bird and Rieker 2008). As Spenner, Otto, and Call (1982, 2) note, "Employment biographies are in part structured by preexisting career lines and the regimes of opportunity that they contain." Within these "regimes of opportunity," however, aides actively construct the caring self, in part by framing their own motivations in terms of personality traits and innate ability.

Even though the career trajectories of home care aides bear clear markings of structural inequality, one positive by-product of years of care work is the emotional capital that accrues over time. Emotional capital provides aides with skills to relate emotionally to clients, in circumstances that are often demanding and stressful. Aides tend to view their relational skills as innate rather than learned, but see them as important job assets nonetheless. Although emotional capital is culturally and socially devalued and doesn't easily translate into social, economic, or cultural capital (Reay 2004), aides and clients alike benefit when workers have strong relational skills. Aides feel better equipped to meet the psychosocial needs of clients after years of providing care and companionship to others. They also achieve a certain sense of dignity knowing that they possess interpersonal skills that others do not have. Clients also benefit from aides' emotional capital. In a field where there is little formal training, aides with established career lines possess learned emotional skills. While these skills may not be formally recognized by the long-term care industry, or even by aides themselves, relational skills help instill dignity in the working lives of aides and reinforce the notion that certain people simply "have what it takes" with respect to caregiving.

Service to Others

The second type of identity work that helps construct the caring self is *service to others*. Aides emphasize their altruistic motivations and downplay their needs for remuneration, while stressing that service to others improves client well-being and their own self-worth. As with other forms of identity talk, many home care workers frame service to others in religious terms, viewing caregiving as "God's work." Each of these narrative strategies further reinforces the caring self in a society that undervalues and undercompensates the work that aides do.

A common theme in aides' talk of service is the notion that their caregiving provides for the unmet needs of elderly and disabled. Aides suggest directly and indirectly that, without their care, clients would be left to suffer alone or in a nursing facility. As such, aides frame their care as making a real difference to the lives of others. José asserts that it is the "little things" he does for his clients that make a sizable difference in their quality of life. He serves his clients by listening to their stories and dignifying them with a little makeup or brush of the hair:

> I can sit there and they'll show me pictures and, "Wow, man!" Early 1900s, you know. I say, "Is that you?" They'll say, "Yeah." "Wow, what a beautiful lady," you know? And then it brightens their day. I love working with women. I had clients that, all I had was women, and I would carry around my own little carrier with the makeup and all sorts of stuff, and I'd make my women pretty. I'd make them pretty, and it made such a difference in them when they would look in the mirror after I was done and bring a smile to their face. And when I'd bring them out, boy, you know, everybody would say, "Oh there goes José's girls."

Shelly, for her part, explains that she learned early in her career that she had the power to "make a difference" in clients' lives. The positive feelings associated with helping others was the prime reason Shelly pursued a career as a nursing assistant:

> It was like 2001 to be exact when I got my STNA [state tested nursing assistant] license. I kept volunteering for Happy Times and I found it really rewarding. Then I went and volunteered at a place called The Meadows, which is for Alzheimer's and dementia. It just so awesome to feel as though you were making a difference. It was just amazing. I actually started as a housekeeper there, and then got my nursing aide license through them.

Although she acknowledges the low pay, commenting that she could make more money at Walmart, Shelly likes "making a connection with these people, changing their lives." Aides like Shelly are empowered by the belief that they are altering people's lives for the better, although it is not always easy to maintain this belief in light of popular conceptions of home care work as "dirty" and home care workers as unreliable and unscrupulous. Virginia is one caregiver who remains strong in her conviction that aides make a difference in the lives of others, despite unflattering stereotypes about the work:

> We all have our pride, but I think when you go into this kind of thing you can't say to yourself, "Hey, I'm in somebody else's bathroom." I mean, I'm

doing things that are meaningful to them. They may seem a little demean-
ing, but it's all part of what you're giving back. And when they [the clients]
trust you,... you're like family to them too, you know?

Virginia's faith in the value of care work extends beyond her own situation. She has confidence and takes pride in the profession as a whole. During our interview, Virginia told of an aide who recently rescued a client
trapped in a burning home. In her retelling of the incident, it was clear
that Virginia felt intense pride and solidarity with the aide, but also a degree of frustration that the public was surprised by the aide's commitment
to her client:

We all get a bad reputation from those that have done bad things during the course of being an aide. But not all aides are like that, and if they
knew.... There was one that was written up in our newspaper. She went
in and she saved her patient from a fire, and I guess the family too. And
I just thought, I am so proud of you. The way the paper read, it was like
they were surprised. I wrote a letter to the gal that did it, and I said,
"You know, I don't know why people are surprised that we would do
that; that's our family." You know, they're like your right leg. What do
you think, you're going to let them burn? You know what I mean? It's
not just about taking advantage of somebody or mistreating them like
you hear.

Like Virginia, many aides perceive their work as stigmatized, either because the work itself is "dirty" or because those who do the work are seen
by the general public as unskilled, thieving, or irresponsible. The social
stigma associated with home care work poses a challenge to the caring self
aides wish to cultivate on the job. Aides engage in identity talk, particularly service to others, as one way of distancing themselves from a population of unprincipled workers, real or imagined.

Another strategy employed by aides to reinforce the caring self and
fend off occupational stigma is to emphasize how service to the elderly
and disabled allows clients to stay at home instead of being placed in an
institution. Tammy, for instance, believes that, without her care, two of her
elderly female clients would be in a nursing home. She tells me, "A big part
of my job is making it possible for Marnie and Kate to stay home as long
as they can." Dawn, similarly, draws a great deal of satisfaction from the

knowledge that aides are necessary and important to people who prefer to convalesce at home:

> I get great satisfaction out of what I do. That's the only reason I'm still in it. Because there's no money in it. There are no benefits to it. But without me—this is going to sound really conceited—but without me or people like me, most of them cannot stay at home.

Dot, of Middletown, has experienced the importance of her role first-hand. She told me of an elderly client, new to her caseload, who had fallen in the night and broken her nose. The client, Farrah, lay on the floor of her apartment, unable to reach the phone, until Dot arrived the next morning. While Dot was horrified that Farrah had been alone for nearly twelve hours, the client repeatedly thanked Dot for arriving when she did. Dot cites this story as one of the reasons she stays in home care, even though she never pictured herself doing such work, envisioning instead a life in retail like the rest of her sisters. As she explains, serving others is the reason why she remains an aide: "I didn't realize how many people need care. Like she [Farrah] said, 'I don't know what I would have done if you weren't here.' It's like, helping people. Being helpful."

Not surprisingly, identity talk that invokes service to others often calls on religious language and belief. Some aides, for example, use religion to describe a kind of conversion experience that propelled them into home care. Early in her career Virginia took a job helping a nun run a respite care program for parents of severely developmentally delayed children. The children were looked after in a facility run by a Catholic church in Middletown, and it was Virginia's job to tend to the children and lead them in religious song and prayer. She recalls an experience directing the children to sing "Jesus Loves Me":

> It was like a miracle in that room. I mean, even though it was impossible to get through with the "Jesus Loves Me," the faces, the look on the faces. And that little blind girl, I'll never forget her face. Just a big smile every time she'd sing it, you know. It was so awesome, and I remember I was so tickled when they said we could take them out, because my son got involved and some of his friends around that age came with us. We took them for ice cream; we'd go to the church across the street. I eventually graduated with my STNA license and people kept asking me, "How can you come back

and not be depressed?" And I say, "If you saw the love." I saw so many miracles in the facility, just somebody taking the time to just be with them.

Moved as she was by these early experiences working with disabled children, Virginia eventually settled on caring for the elderly in home settings, seeking a job with greater relational autonomy. Nonetheless, she claims that time spent in the Catholic facility "converted" her to care work. Other aides couch their identity talk in religious terms to draw attention to their high standards of care. Kristen, for example, feels that her religious background not only directs her into caregiving, as we learned earlier, but that it motivates her to provide care with integrity:

> I don't know if I would act with integrity if I wasn't a Christian, but I am a Christian and it sure does help. I'll come in [the client's house], and she'll say, "Oh honey, there's nothing to do today." I say, "There has to be something to do today. That's why I'm here."

Lete, a caregiver who recently emigrated from Mexico, calls on traditional Christian teaching to explain why she is willing to work as an aide even though the pay is low and the work conditions often tough: "I've always wanted to do something like this. There must be something else than paying the bills, making money. I have a lot of love when I look at them [the clients]. I see Christ in them. I'm working for God." As Lete's identity talk suggests, aides often position serving others in opposition to making money, as though the two are incompatible. Lete uses explicit religious language to play up her altruistic motivations, while other nonreligious aides use less devout frames of reference. Either way, home care aides engage in identity talk about compensation to assure themselves and others that they are "not in it for the money," a key narrative component of the caring self. One caregiver explains the lack of financial motivation in this way: "The money is fine, but I'm just not in it for the money. I really can't explain it. It's more than money. Money can't pay what I have to give. There's not enough money, you know?" And Mark, from Central City, agrees that money is but a small motivating factor in his care work: "It's not so much the money, although the money helps you live. It's called—what's the reward? The reward is actually, how good do you feel about yourself and what have you done for the day?"

Like most of us, Mark seeks job satisfaction and a kind of reward that is not just monetary. He expresses minor annoyance that he is paid nine dollars an hour to care for six different clients, each for minimal hours, without access to benefits or career advancement (not to mention that he travels from client to client on bicycle, averaging—he estimates—thirty miles a day). Mark is undoubtedly living among the ranks of the working poor in Central City, where the cost of living is relatively high. Even so, Mark achieves a sense of dignity and pride at work, his caring self, by engaging in identity talk that highlights his altruistic, rather than financial, interests in care work.

Unlike Mark, some caregivers are more candid about their struggles to make ends meet. Even in these instances, however, the identity talk of serving others provides a compelling narrative for aides. Sandra, a white home care worker in her midforties, cares for several clients in Central City. When I ask her to comment on the wages she receives in exchange for her care, she replies:

> Okay. You know somebody's got to do it, and you know you're not going to get paid beaucoup bucks. I feel it takes somebody special to be in this line of work. Not everybody can do it. It's like my daughter said, "Momma, I could never do it." I look at it in the aspect that I'm helping that person get better. I have a part in that. So it's real, it's self-rewarding.

Sandra's comment that it is "self-rewarding" to aid a person as they heal physically and emotionally suggests that, beyond altruism, serving others can be mutually beneficial for aides and clients. Indeed, the reciprocal benefits of serving others figures centrally in the identity talk of aides, who draw attention to the shared benefits that come from caring for a dependent person.

Lete, as we learned earlier, works for an elderly woman with whom she has a loving but stressful relationship. She acknowledges that the emotional strain takes a toll but Lete remains committed to the client because "it [caregiving] makes you feel good, like nothing else." Similarly, Mary describes her emotional state when she arrives at work to care for her elderly client, Rose: "She makes me feel alive when I walk in the door." Fahima, an aide originally from Belize who now lives in Central City, describes something similar as her motivation for paid caregiving:

> When I close this door at night behind me, I feel good being home because I know I had accomplished something because there was somebody that I

helped along the way.... The priority for me is giving them what I could give them. Which is what I call my all-in-all. That's what I do.

As each of these accounts shows, service to others is a salient part of the identity talk that aides engage in while constructing the caring self. The point here is not that home care aides are all saints driven by altruistic impulses. Rather, home care workers clearly feel compelled to engage in altruistic identity talk as part of a broader need to construct a caring self. Given the stigmatized nature of the work and popular beliefs that home care aides are unskilled, unmotivated, or deceitful, it should come as little surprise that workers would proactively narrate their care as a service that benefits themselves, their clients, and society more generally. Professing a service to others, however, is not enough to secure the caring self. Aides must also demonstrate that their altruistic motivations sit in stark contrast to the apathy of "uncaring others," including families, agencies, doctors, and other home care aides.

Boundary Making Above and Below

In constructing the caring self, aides tout their abilities to provide for clients while drawing attention to the shortcomings of "uncaring others." In so doing, aides engage in identity talk that draws clear boundaries "above and below" (Lamont 2000). As Michele Lamont (2000) notes in her book on working-class men, "boundary work" allows social actors of low socioeconomic status to achieve a sense of dignity and moral worth by "constructing similarities and differences between themselves and other groups" (3). In the context of home care, aides emphasize their superior caregiving skills relative to family members and doctors (boundary making above) and relative to other paid caregivers (boundary making below).

As they draw boundaries "above," aides often reference the hands-on, personal care they provide for clients. The term "personal care" is a somewhat euphemistic term for the less savory tasks associated with paid care work: changing diapers, cleaning catheters, bathing or showering clients, cleaning teeth or dentures, attending to necrotic tissue, and other similar tasks. Home care aides are quick to speak about how little personal care bothers them, aware that most people perceive the work to be "dirty." Sophie, for example, talks nonchalantly about her quadriplegic client, whose bowel she routinely "scrapes." When asked how she feels about the task, Sophie delights in describing this particular form of personal care: "I can do anything. She [the client] had no bowel movement. It stayed in the lower part of the bowel, so I had to take it out. She was not able to pass, so you have to, with gloves on, scrape it out."

As Sophie's narrative suggests, it is not uncommon for this sort of "dirty work" to become routine, and to even be a source of pride, for the person doing it. Research in medical sociology suggests that all medical providers attempt to regulate, bureaucratize, and routinize those things that are considered traumatic or aberrant life events to the rest of us (Chambliss 1996; Katz Rothman 1983; Roth 1963). However, in contrast to Daniel Chambliss's (1996) findings that hospital nurses seek ways to make routine and "profane" those tasks unthinkable to most of us, home care aides go to great lengths to demonstrate how "sacred" the profane act of bathing or grooming can be. Workers emphasize the dirty part of their work as a way of drawing boundaries between themselves and others, simultaneously fortifying the caring self.

Jackie is one aide who speaks with absolute confidence about her talent for bathing clients:

> Let me make this note. When I go in there—I'm going to tell you, if you ever meet one of my clients, they would tell you, I give them the best bath, shower. Even the men. Everybody do not know how to give a bath. I wish I could teach them how.

Jackie goes on to say that her clients often brag to the agency about her personal care skills. In partial jest, she adds that she is so good that family and friends who don't need home care have requested her services. Jackie takes great pride in her care of elderly clients and distinguishes herself from aides who avoid personal care: "A lot of them [caregivers] don't like to do it. I had to train a girl on how to shower one day. And I don't think they like doing it. I don't like my patients to smell. I don't like that."

José, too, believes it is important to pay attention to personal care, for both the client's well-being and his own job satisfaction. He notes that the kind of personal care he provides is something aides working in facilities cannot offer:

> My men, I don't like to see my men with any kind of, you know, shabby looking beards. Sometimes I had a gentleman that might want to grow a beard. "That's okay, you can grow it, but we're going to keep it trimmed. The minute I see that it ain't working, it's coming off. We don't want you looking shabby." It just

made a difference to all of them, you know. I mean their personal care. It's just hygiene, getting them dressed every day in something different. It could still be clean and I would say, "No, I want to put something different on you today." That's what they need because it's something that they used to be able to do but they can no longer do it. A lot of places, the workers don't have the time.

Katy, a woman in her midsixties who identifies as Filipino and white, is nearing retirement after thirty years of working as an aide. She talks with great appreciation for the workings of the body:

> You know, families don't cope well with it [personal care]. It [urine and excrement] gets into the couch and those kinds of things, then I come over and clean it up....It didn't seem odd to me. That's what older people do. It's about knowing that, for an old person, when you cough, you wet your pants. Wonderful. It's wonderful.

Katy, like many other caregivers, sharpens the contrast between herself on the one hand and families who "don't cope" on the other. It is not uncommon to hear aides assert their expertise by drawing a boundary between themselves and family members who are absent, incompetent, or who "just don't care." Instead of *distancing* themselves from potentially stigmatizing "dirty work," aides emphasize their own aptitude for such duties and their willingness to perform them.

Aides' construction of boundaries between themselves and "uncaring" family extend well beyond the realm of personal care. Busy families or those who live far from an elderly or disabled relative must rely on aides to provide the bulk of care, physical and emotional. Paid caregivers are often critical of families who care for a loved one at arm's length, carrying quiet judgments about absent or busy relatives. At times, aides become frustrated with choices that families make, especially when those choices appear to jeopardize clients' best interests or quality of life. Fahima remembers fighting to keep one of her clients, an elderly woman with Alzheimer's, off medication and out of a nursing home. Unable to persuade the family to keep the client at home, Fahima draws clear boundaries between what she thinks is best for her client and the family's decision to institutionalize:

> You tried to take her [the client] for a walk, she's so sleepy. Her knees start wobbling; you got to turn back and take her back home. I say, "This is not

working." Daughter says, "Well, that's okay. We'll put her in a home." They put her in a wheelchair and that was it. She never walked again. She never walked again. I say, "This is going to be the end of her." And she says, "I don't think so." She died. It's just that they believed whatever the doctor says is gospel.

Due to their proximity to clients, aides feel they have a better grasp of clients' immediate needs than distant family members do. Other aides make clear that they have skills and talents that others do not have, simply because of the time spent on the front lines of care: "Sometimes even the family don't really know because they're not really in it. They just maybe take care of the mom or whoever is sick. But they really don't know because not everyone is *gifted* to do it." Maureen, a white caregiver, recalls her concern about the way a former client, who she called "grandma," was treated by a daughter. The boundary drawn between Maureen and the uncaring daughter serves to underscore Maureen's superior position as the caring member of a "fictive kin" network:

> She [Grandma] would smile when I came in. When her granddaughter would come in, and the kids, I'd always bring them and talk with her, you know. And the daughter would come in and make some kind of comment. Grandma would just kind of roll her eyes.... She knew that her daughter was uncaring.

Similarly, Dot, from Middletown, recounts a time that she was asked to drive one of her elderly clients, Jewel, to a relative's house two miles down the street. The family member, a granddaughter, was the only relative living close by, yet Dot had not seen or met her in a year of providing care to Jewel. Dot struggles to understand homes where "there's no family structure" and makes clear that her own sick and elderly relatives are cared for by a slew of family, including herself. Even though Dot makes a living filling the "care gap" for other families, she is unequivocal that paid caregivers would never be employed in her own family.

Shelly, also working in Middletown, is equally disdainful of families who fail to meet what she sees as familial caring obligations. She makes sharp the contrast between herself and family members who "disappear" when real care is needed, only to show up after a client passes:

> Everybody with Alzheimer's and dementia, a lot of their family members forget that they're even there. So we are those people's neighbors and

friends; they call us if they have a problem. They don't call their kids. And I still look back and say, "Why do they care now that she's passed away?" They didn't care when she wasn't getting her meds. They didn't care when she didn't have briefs. They didn't care when she didn't have laundry, or soap, to do her dishes.

Knowing a client's needs intimately translates into caregivers' sense of expertise and moral authority in relation to the medical community as well. Home care workers are clearly at the bottom of the medical hierarchy but are quick to claim jurisdiction over client care. They do this in part through boundary work that characterizes medical professionals as busy, uncaring, and cold, and aides as attentive and emotionally engaged. Camilla, from Central City, expresses her feelings in this way:

When you're a CNA, that's the bottom they say. But you spend more time with the clients. And that's why I'll stay a CNA for a while, because with the other ones—LVNs and RNs and so on—they do a lot of paperwork. They don't spend their life with people. They don't know. They come to the CNAs to ask about the patient, because they don't know. I'm like the number-one person. I spend a majority of the time with them.

Katy feels that she has never been respected around doctors, especially when she worked in a convalescent home. Katy now refuses to work in skilled nursing facilities because of the poor working conditions and treatment of patients. After complaining to a doctor about the treatment of elderly clients in a convalescent home where she last worked, Katy quit and never returned:

You know, nobody'll listen to you. They just say, "Yeah, yeah, yeah, you're the aides." I get so tired of being thought of as incompetent and stupid and that I don't know anything. I think it's always been that way and it will continue to be that way. But we're the ones who know the patients. But it's the power trip, the control trip [on the part of doctors]. But I could care less and I do what I do.

We can tell from this account that Katy feels some frustration about being disrespected by doctors, but is able to reassert the caring self by insisting that she is the one who "really knows" patients. This grounded knowledge preserves aides' dignity and sense of self at work, and empowers them to make assessments about patient health that come from years of hands-on experience. Fahima, discussing a client for whom she works, expresses concern about the way that doctors rely on quick fixes and medications without thinking about the implications for patient quality of life:

> She [the client] was unable to do anything for herself. And I tell them [the doctors], "You have to let her try for herself." If you keep them on all this medication and just let them sleep and don't try to exercise them, you won't get anything other than—they are going to waste away. They are not able to help themselves, so you have to help them.

Fahima's comments support Everett Hughes's (1971, 344) observation that workers at the bottom of a work hierarchy believe themselves in possession of a "magical power" that comes from saving a person of more acknowledged skill—like a doctor—from his or her own mistakes. Most caregivers express, as part of their identity work, a deep belief that their care either prevented an unwanted medical intervention and possible medical error, or helped mitigate the damage of physician intervention. In those instances when physicians disregarded or failed to solicit aides' firsthand knowledge, aides reasserted their value by playing up their intimate knowledge of clients' physical and emotional needs, positioning themselves against what they characterize as the arrogance or indifference of physicians.

In addition to drawing boundaries "above" with clients' families and doctors, aides create distinctions "below." Like the working-class men in Lamont's *Dignity of Working Men* (2000), home care aides engage in boundary work to distance themselves from less conscientious workers, their colleagues in the field whom they portray as less professional, reliable, or caring about their work. Even though rates of physical elder abuse in paid home care are very low relative to abuse at the hands of informal family caregivers (National Center on Elder Abuse 1998), workers speak at length about other aides who "just don't care" or who "give the rest of us a bad reputation." These narratives are fueled by sensationalized stories in the press, such as the case of the aide in California who committed double suicide with his client.[2] In distancing themselves from "bad" workers, aides blame the agencies for making poor hiring decisions, while also condemning workers who demonstrate a weak work ethic.

Andrew believes that the agencies in particular make poor hiring decisions, allowing "uneducated" men and women into the field, although he concedes that things have improved since workers in Central City received a wage increase:

> Now they pay more so you can get more professional people in this kind of work.... Back then, it was people on drugs, people who were alcoholics, and they were hiring them off the streets. So a person come in and they steal from you, break into houses later, and take stuff. Now you get much more quality. Some of the people are much more educated. I mean, I have a high school diploma, and I have some years of trying to learn, and stuff like that. But many of them, they don't have that. Eighth grade, you know?

Several workers have witnessed instances of other aides quitting with little notice, sleeping on the job, or failing to complete the most basic caregiving tasks. Recounting stories of unconscientious workers, aides express frustration that their peers fail to meet basic ethical and moral standards of care. Dot, for example, is angry when aides quit without giving advance notice to the agency. Although such actions do not directly affect Dot, she worries about the consequences for clients when a worker fails to show up. In her mind, "quitters" fail to recognize the importance of caring for another human being:

> What frustrates me more than anything is people that would work and then just call off and quit and not give notice. It really frustrates me because it's like, "We're not working in a factory, people, where there's somebody there all the time. You're taking care of a person. And you just can't up and quit like that."

More commonly, aides find fault with other workers' on-the-job performance. Although aides rarely work in teams, clients who require around-the-clock care employ multiple caregivers to meet their needs. In these circumstances, aides frequently overlap shifts or see one another before or after a shift change, which gives them the opportunity to observe one another. Many of the aides in the sample are over the age of fifty (a number of them are over sixty), and they posit that age strongly determines work ethic. Mary, sixty-seven, works with several aides in their early twenties and claims that "they [the younger aides] just don't want to work. They don't want to do anything. They just sit there." Virginia, sixty-two, agrees: "It seems like the older women seem a little more feet-on-the-ground. They know how to do a toilet, how to clean a refrigerator, how not to be on the cell phone." Virginia had a recent confrontation with another aide caring for her client, Tally. Virginia would often arrive at Tally's apartment to find the aide, thirty-five years Virginia's junior, sleeping on the couch. In addition to witnessing such things firsthand, Virginia has also heard countless stories of impropriety over the years. She laments that, because of the actions of a few unscrupulous aides, home care workers as a whole are regarded as less trustworthy and are given less responsibility:

> Over the years I've heard so many stories about stuff. And it went through phases with people being ripped off, things stolen. And we used to be able to take them to the bank. We used to be able to go and take the check for them, like a personal check, to go in and get the groceries and stuff. But I don't even think we're allowed to do that.

Kristen, sixty-five, was very vocal during our interview about "incompetent" aides she has encountered. While supervising the care of her own aunt, Kristen helped hire a young aide for a few hours a week so that she could continue working as a home care aide herself. After two weeks, Kristen learned that her aunt's aide was "hiding" during most of her shift at the Laundromat across the street, ostensibly washing clothes. The aide would often leave her shift without checking in with Kristen's aunt, abandoning clothes midcycle. Kristen is furious that aides of such low caliber are employed by agencies and that they remain on the job even after repeated complaints about their behavior.

Actual misconduct of aides is certainly disturbing, and when it occurs, it seems to confirm to the public the suspicion that home care workers are unskilled, unreliable, and sometimes unethical. Although I never directly witnessed the neglect, benign or otherwise, of clients at the hands of aides, there is little reason to doubt the accounts relayed by Kristen, Dot, and Virginia. Other aides in the study, including younger workers, public health nurses, and agency administrators, also alluded to, albeit in vague terms, the problem of "bad" caregivers. Positioned on the front lines of care, aides are certainly well positioned to observe both minor and egregious breaches of conduct.

When aides act in uncaring ways toward clients, the caring self is potentially undermined for other workers. For this reason, it is imperative that aides incorporate "bad" aides into their identity talk, thereby distancing themselves from any stigma by association, or what Goffman (1963) calls "courtesy stigma." Just as aides draw boundaries between themselves and the family members and physicians they regard as uncaring, they also separate themselves from dishonest or lazy aides. These boundaries, crucial to identity talk, allow aides to promote the caring self as an altruistic identity sustained by a deep-seated, natural conviction to care.

Each dimension of identity work outlined above—professing care as natural or innate, valuing a job providing service to others, and drawing boundaries above and below—supports and enables the construction of the caring self. While this talk among aides in the sample varied somewhat by age, all aides, regardless of race, ethnicity, or gender, engaged in similar broad patterns of identity construction. This is not to say that social location is irrelevant to the caring self. On the contrary, race and ethnicity shape aides' construction of the caring self, further indicating a racial division of labor in home care.

Race, Ethnicity, and the Caring Self

All caregivers construct a caring self on the job in an effort to present their care as a socially valuable service, motivated first and foremost by altruism. This general finding holds across age, race, ethnicity, and gender of aide. That said, the caring self varies by race and ethnicity in important ways. Racism on the part of some white clients and agency managers, not to mention other aides, makes the caring self more difficult for aides of color to achieve. In spite of these experiences of racism and discrimination, and perhaps because of it, aides of color engage in identity talk that frames their care work as superior. In this way, paid caregivers engage in boundary work similar to that of the working-class black men in Lamont's (2000) study, professing a caring self superior to that of whites.

Half of the aides interviewed for the book were nonwhite. The sub-sample includes two Asian Americans, two Asians who are not yet U.S. citizens, five Latinos (two of whom are U.S. citizens), six African Americans, and one aide who identified herself as half white, half Filipino. Nine of the sixteen are foreign born. All of the aides in this group experienced some form of on-the-job discrimination or racism, usually at the hands of an elderly or disabled client. In these moments, race and ethnicity became salient factors in their work lives.

With few exceptions, aides of color spoke of "incidents" where they were accused of stealing something from a client's home. I argue that this is the most significant challenge to worker dignity, precisely because client distrust destroys the narrative foundation of the caring self, that is, the belief that caregivers are altruistically motivated. An accusation of stealing, especially when tinged with racism, is an emotional experience for aides, who then feel betrayed and undermined by the very people for whom they care. Aides of color, African American aides in particular, appear more susceptible to charges of stealing relative to aides who are white. Although it is difficult to draw definitive conclusions from such a small sample, African American aides are unequivocal in the their beliefs that race (or racism) is a factor when white clients accuse them of stealing.

Camilla, an African American caregiver from Central City, has worked in home care for several years and could recall countless incidents of discrimination. She is not always certain whether racism is at play, like the time her client suddenly requested a different aide "for no reason." But other instances leave little doubt.

Camilla's clients are mostly white, African American, and Latino. She says she finds "Hispanics" the most welcoming to her and whites to be the least so, although she reminds me that she has amiable relationships with most of her clients. During our nearly two-hour lunch conversation, Camilla talked about a series of "run-ins" she had with elderly white clients. In 1991, Camilla was offered a job caring for a Russian woman in a suburb of Central City. The position required heavy cleaning, so Camilla was offered nearly ten dollars an hour, six dollars above the minimum wage at the time. Jumping at the opportunity, she arrived at Olga's house early her first day on the job and rang the doorbell. The woman answered and appeared visibly unsettled, but Camilla reassured her that she was there to help dress and bathe her, as well as to do some cleaning in the house. Olga refused to let Camilla enter, demanding instead that she remain outside to "fix up the yard." Since tending the yard was not part of the job description, Camilla asked to be let into the house. Growing agitated, Olga ordered Camilla to "say nothing" and do the work outside. Conceding, Camilla returned to her car and drove to the nearest pay phone to alert her manager to the situation. The manager, sympathetic to Camilla, told her to wait patiently while he found "another girl" to help out.

Nearly an hour later, a white aide turned up, someone with whom Camilla had a cordial working relationship. After greeting the new aide, Olga let both women into her home and then watched as they divided the cleaning labor, Camilla in the kitchen and the other aide in the living room. As Camilla worked, she observed Olga chatting pleasantly with the white aide, asking questions about her family, and about whether she would like a root beer or coffee. No such pleasantries were exchanged with Camilla, who realized that racism was clearly guiding the woman's social interaction. Although Camilla agreed to return to Olga's house a second time with her colleague, she then asked to be reassigned. Even though the money was good, she felt too humiliated to even go to work. As she put it, "I'm leaving.... My thing is, if you come at me with that racist stuff, I'm outta here. I'm out! Good-bye."

Camilla recalls other situations involving more "subtle" forms of racism. She describes being "tested" by the wife of an elderly client, who feared Camilla was stealing from them:

> I took care of this older white man years ago. His wife tried to set me up. She would go out to the store. I was coming in to give him a shower and dress him. I'd give her time to go out and do her grocery shopping. Well, what would she do? She would take his money in his wallet, right out there. The money be on top of the wallet. And you know how people paper clip their money to see if someone take their money? I said, "Okay!" Then I told my boss, this lady is doing this. And she did it again. But after that time, I guess she realized I wasn't going to take her money.

Feeling surveilled was common for aides of color, who were keenly aware of the various tactics clients employed to prevent theft. Jackie, an African American aide from Central City, is sympathetic to elderly clients who feel the need to keep tabs on aides, even though she feels some of the precautions are extreme. Several of her clients, for example, have "little cameras around" to observe her behavior, something that she reluctantly accepts: "They [the clients] get really frightened because of something that has happened, or different things on TV, and maybe because someone has come into their home and taken things."

Like Camilla and Jackie, Andrew has worked for clients of many different races and ethnicities. He has experienced racism from all clients, including African Americans who were "disappointed" that he was black. He is simultaneously conscious of and sanguine about the racism that confronts him at work, even if that means dealing with clients' lack of trust:

> It is very important that you always program yourself, when you go in another person's house. You're in that person's house and you're caring for that person. Your personal feelings have to be kind of like pushed aside, because you're dealing with quite a lot of things. You're dealing with people from all different walks of life, people from all different races, religions. Sometimes we're called things that we don't like, but you know, you have to push them to the side. I'm making a living. The most important thing with clients is that they're able to trust you. Because I've been in many homes where, you know, they'll leave fifty or sixty dollars laying around to see if I would take it.

Fahima, from Central City, also has learned to deal with clients who display a lack of trust. While clearly affronted by accusations of stealing, something she has encountered "on more than one occasion," Fahima would not leave her job because of it. In the end, her motivation to care—and reinforce the caring self—trumps any indignation that comes from false accusations:

> It's the medication speaking, not him [the client]. Just let it go past and go on. And move on. Because otherwise you would have to pick up your purse and walk right through the door and don't even look back. But you can't do that.

It is important to note that none of the white aides, in either city, talked about being surveilled or mistrusted by their clients. As mentioned earlier, it is difficult to draw definitive conclusions given the sample size, but in this study aides of color appear more susceptible to charges of stealing relative to aides who are white. Among nonwhite aides, African Americans report experiencing more racism than aides who are Latino or of Asian descent. This reality does not escape the attention of some of the white aides, especially younger ones, who have heard about or experienced a client's racism toward minority groups. Shelly, a white aide, recently asked to be transferred from a white client living in Middletown because of her racist attitudes toward African Americans. Initially, she "adored" the client, a woman in her eighties, but soon tired of her "derogatory" language about blacks, specifically, her statements that they were lazy and criminal. After hearing the "n-word" several times from her client, Shelly asked to be reassigned. Commenting on her decision to leave, she says, "Opinions—everybody's entitled to them. Unfortunately, I don't impose mine on you; you shouldn't impose yours on me." Soon after leaving the case, Shelly received a phone call from the client's son, who blamed her for his mother's death just days earlier, citing the stress of their disagreement about race. Undeterred by the son's accusation, Shelly made it known to her manager that she would no longer provide care to clients who espouse racist beliefs.

Although this incident had the potential to undermine Shelly's caring self, given that she ultimately chose to leave her client on short notice, it is also clear that Shelly's work identity is safely intact. As a white woman never directly subjected to racial discrimination by clients, Shelly has little to lose by taking the moral high ground on the issue of race. In contrast, aides like Andrew, Camilla, and Jackie must carefully decide when and how to object to racism, since they are regularly exposed to both overt and subtle forms of discrimination. Quite simply, it would be impractical for aides of color to request reassignment each time they were subjected to this type of abuse. Additionally, nonwhite aides feel collectively under suspicion because of their race, something that serves to undermine the caring self over time. As Feagin and Sikes (1994, 16–17) suggest, racism for African Americans is experienced in a cumulative way—many instances over many years—and can significantly affect one's behavior and life perspective. I suggest that aides of color experience racism on the job as potential assaults to their caring selves and must be strategic about their responses to these experiences. As discussed previously, aides of color do recognize and name racism and discrimination in their lives, but are fairly resigned about whites' behavior, insisting that the best response is to "push feelings aside" or "move on."

Cultural Difference and the Caring Self

Even though racism and discrimination challenge the caring selves of certain aides, particularly the African American men and women interviewed, certain forms of identity talk help these and other aides bolster their workplace identities. In addition to engaging in broad forms of identity talk common to all aides, aides of color commonly frame their caring dispositions in terms of racial or ethnic difference. This seems especially true for caregivers who are nonnatives of the United States. In contrast, most white aides are hesitant to talk about caregiving in terms of race or ethnicity, although a small number spoke in explicitly racist ways about nonwhite caregivers.

In cases where the caregiver is an immigrant to the United States, cultural difference is used to explain the intense devotion to clients and reinforce the caring self. As documented by Ehrenreich and Hochschild (2002), Parrenas (2001), and Diamond (1992), care labor is increasingly the work of immigrant women who take paid positions in the United States tending to children or elderly clients, while their own families remain at home or in their country of origin. Consistent with these earlier findings, immigrant aides in the study spoke of separations from family while caring for someone else's parent or spouse. At the same time, these aides emphasized their capacity for care work, noting that cultural difference predisposes them to the job.

Hannah and George, two Filipino aides, recently immigrated to the United States after spending the previous ten years working as registered nurses in the Philippines. The married couple are sponsored by a for-profit care company that arranges for foreign caregivers to receive work visas in exchange for contracted employment with an agency for a minimum of three years. The couple have two children at home in the Philippines, cared for by their grandparents. Although Hannah and George feel homesick and are somewhat unhappy about being demoted to the position of nursing aide, both believe the move to the United States will benefit the family in the long term. They also see themselves as possessing an expertise and orientation to care unique to Filipino workers. As George describes it:

We work good. We are very industrious. We don't mind working whenever and for how long. Anything goes. We have that thing, that if you're being paid, just work. We don't mind, after eight hours, if there are tasks that need to be done, then we want to finish it.

Katy, an aide from Central City, has strong established beliefs about caregivers from the Philippines. Herself mixed-race Filipina and white, Katy's obvious admiration for Filipino aides seems to have little to do with her own identity or heritage and more to do with her observations of other aides on the job. She tells me:

Filipino workers are the best ones I've ever seen. I told my sister, if I get sick, I want a Filipino. They are just very mellow. They are very caring. The men are very caring and very, very good, too. They have been my favorite caregivers to work with, the male Filipino caregivers. And they are still a little subservient and afraid.

In contrast to Filipinos, Katy offers the observation that Somali, Korean, and Chinese caregivers are "not good," although she finds it difficult to elaborate when pressed for details. Having completed a short training course on cultural diversity early in her career, Katy seemed most animated when talking about racial and ethnic variations among clients. She spoke at length about one of her clients, a South Asian woman, who was paralyzed on her right side. Katy explained that because Indian custom is to eat with your right hand and "take care of your body" with your left, her client refused to eat in front of anyone since she relied exclusively on her left hand. Crediting her training course, Katy felt equipped to attend to this woman with different cultural beliefs. When I asked her to elaborate on whether those cultural differences extend to caregivers, Katy unequivocally agreed and offered the following summary:

Filipinos have three washcloths. One for your face, one for your body, and one for your bottom. Do not mix them up! It's interesting what you learn along the way. And the Mexican aides—they are very particular about washing the inside of their [clients'] thighs.

Michael, a Chinese American who immigrated to the United States nearly ten years ago, feels that his ethnic heritage is central to his work, especially when he cares for elderly Chinese living in Central City. Michael believes that the Chinese Americans in the city are basically "out of luck" because so few medical and social service providers speak Mandarin. He sees himself as providing desperately needed, culturally competent services that his clients would not otherwise receive. Each day, for example, Michael travels to the small Chinatown in Central City to care for an elderly Chinese American woman, Mai, who has cancer. Michael ensures that Mai receives a traditional herbal remedy that helps ease the side effects of chemotherapy, something her U.S. doctors have dismissed:

> I encourage her to take herbs. I just cook her up some.... My experience is that American doctors are normally not that sensitive. They don't believe in herbs, you know, because they've never tried it. I think generally American doctors are willing to help, but to a certain degree they're pretty naive about how the medicine, the Asian medicine, the herbs, could help the body.

Fahima, originally from Belize, also suggests that her cultural background influences her caregiving sensibilities, especially her tendencies to respect elders and get along with others:

> You know the expression "It takes a village"? I was raised in a different culture, and I tell them that my parents taught us, "You must learn to live with an aunt," and if you can live with an aunt, you can live with anybody. Because believe me, some of them are not easy to get along with. But you just got to look past that.

Aides of color born in the United States express similar sentiments about their talents for respecting and getting along with others, although they do not attribute their ability to cultural, racial, or ethnic difference. Instead, a color-blind philosophy that downplays difference and emphasizes what people have in common underpins their personal narratives. Jackie, an African American aide, is resolute that race does not matter for caregiving, even though she has experienced client racism on more than one occasion. She insists, "You [the client] may be a little bit lighter, maybe a little bit darker; we're just one." Andrew, like Jackie, invokes a similar color blindness to make sense of his daily interactions with whites, while at the same time making it clear that he is fully aware of racial differences. Andrew describes his work with white clients as something that enhances his personal and professional growth:

> Most of my clients are white, you know, and it's like we establish, we don't even see the color barrier anymore. It's a special feeling, you know. And Bert, and all of them, I learned a lot from dealing with other cultures and different backgrounds as well. I learned a tremendous amount about what people think about other people, and their background and race. You learn so much—very educational. It's been quite an experience for me and it's opened up other avenues for me. I mean, I'm venturing out and communicating with people from all different races and walks of life.

In general, white aides also use color-blind language to talk about caregiving, insisting that quality of care has little to do with nationality, race, or ethnicity. Unlike aides of color, however, white aides do not experience racism at the hands of clients and so never have to reconcile their racial identity with the caring self. As a result, white aides' general insistence that race is "not an issue" is less an accurate reflection of racial conditions and more an indication of the way that color-blind ideologies mask the race privilege that white aides experience in the workplace.

A small number of white aides happily offered their views on cultural differences in caregiving, at times using explicitly racial (even racist) language. These few women imply that care work is the domain of white women and that quality of care is adversely affected when women of color do the job. Maureen, a white aide living in Central City, remarks that the occupation attracts large numbers of Latinos, a trend she is not too happy about:

> The money isn't that great, but they [caregivers] need a job, and some of these people.... There are a lot of Spanish speaking. I have nothing against Spanish speaking, but they're Mexican people. I've got nothing against Mexican people, but they're limited on the places where they can work, and they seem to draw the worst kind.

Mary, of Middletown, has a casual work-related friendship with an African American aide, Doreen, with whom she shares care of an elderly client. The aide, according to Mary, "does her job well," a fact that Mary struggles to reconcile with her stereotypes about African Americans as "lazy." She describes Doreen this way:

> She's kind of different than a lot of the black people. She wants to get ahead, it sounds like she has a good husband, and she has two children. It's really helped change my perspective on the black people. She's not like the typical blacks that I think of.... A lot of the black girls don't want to do as much. They just sit there and expect you to do it all.

Mary admits that she doesn't like to work for black *clients* either, a prejudice reinforced last year by a sour relationship with an elderly African American woman, Janey. Describing black clients as "too particular," Mary explains that Janey was "verbally abusive...like I was the slave and she was the master." Though she initially laughs at her own analogy, Mary's mood quickly shifts as she confides that "being put down" by Janey reminded her of the many years she lived with an abusive husband (now an ex-husband). After working a week for Janey, Mary asked to be reassigned and requested she work for white clients from then on.

Maureen and Mary, both older women in their sixties, are in the minority among white workers with respect to their views on race. It is possible (and likely) that other white aides harbor similar views but are simply less candid. That said, most aides—including aides of color—convincingly call on color-blind language to insist that race is a nonissue in caregiving. Observations of cultural difference most commonly emanate from aides born outside the United States, who reference their racial, ethnic, or cultural backgrounds to explain why they do care work and why they do it so well. For these few men and women in the study, talk about cultural differences is another way to give substance to the caring self, allowing aides to ground their propensity to care in long-standing cultural traditions and obligations.

How do these findings fit with structural realities linked to the racial division of paid reproductive labor? As Nakano Glenn (1992) reminds us, women of color have a long history of providing domestic service work, a reality that in part explains their continued occupational subordination and disadvantage in the service sector. This reality has "gone global" as more and more women of color migrate from the global South to the global North to provide child and elder care (Ehrenreich and Hochschild 2002).

The stories of Hannah and George, Fahima, Andrew, Jackie, Camilla, and Michael all reflect to some degree the racialized inequality of low-wage care work. Hannah and George, for example, are contractually bound to an unskilled home care job, for which they are overqualified, in exchange for the promise of citizenship and greater prosperity in the United States. Both have sacrificed ties to their own families to do the work, and their ultimate success likely depends on economic forces out of their control and probably some degree of luck. Andrew, Jackie, and Camilla—all African American—find themselves working for elderly and disabled clients, many of them white. Like the domestic workers given voice in Rollins's (1985) and Romero's (1992) respective works, these three home care aides encounter racism and paternalism serving white clients, in a job that carries little in the way of pecuniary reward. To make sense of these realities, they adopt very frank language about the overt discrimination they've faced, while at the same time using color-blind rhetoric to speak generally about their strong predisposition for the job of caregiving. These realities leave little doubt that home care workers of color, like other domestic workers, provide care in the context of genuine inequality.

Despite the inequalities associated with home care work, aides of all backgrounds find ways to maneuver within structural constraint to find dignity and satisfaction at work. Constructing the caring self—a situated identity formed in daily interaction with clients, families, medical professionals, and agency managers—is central to the way in which aides find meaning in an occupation that is seen by others as "dirty" and that carries minimal extrinsic reward. All the aides I interviewed actively construct the caring self to reinforce their care as natural, altruistic, and better quality than that which is offered by other "uncaring others." In combination with high relational autonomy relative to other service jobs and fictive kinship ties with clients, the caring self enables workers to sustain dignity while caring for their charges. The caring self serves to foster dignity for all aides, irrespective of their race, ethnicity, or gender.

Even as aides of color engage in the same construction of the caring self as white aides, they face clear challenges to this identity formation, mostly in the form of racist clients who question their motivation and intentions. These aides work to reinforce the caring self by downplaying the significance of racist encounters and emphasizing caregiving as a color-blind endeavor. Others play up cultural differences in caregiving as a way of reinforcing the caring self. In these instances, traditions or values from another country or culture are narrated as valued resources that caregivers bring to their work and that predispose them to provide high-quality care.[3] White women, in contrast, either view caregiving as a color-blind endeavor or make note of racial and ethnic differences as a way of distancing themselves from aides of color. Whether aides emphasize or downplay race and culture, the ultimate goal—interactionally speaking—is to maintain the caring self for themselves and others.

Of what consequence is the caring self, sociologically speaking? On both an individual and collective level, the caring self allows home care aides to establish dignity and social worth in an invisible, devalued, and "dirty" job. Aides publicly construct a narrative of work around themes of service and psychosocial reward rather than insufficient pay, job instability, or exploitation (even though, as discussed earlier, these are also realities of the work). In so doing, aides tell an important story about the way that service workers assert agency within an occupational sector that generally disadvantages them, even in jobs characterized by high degrees of emotional labor. To sociologists studying low-waged labor, and interactive service work in particular, such a story affirms that workers can indeed secure dignity and a sense of worth in socially devalued or "tainted" occupations (Ashforth and Kreiner 1999; Ashforth et al. 2007; Drew, Mills, and Gassaway 2007; Hodson 2001; Newman 1999b). An obvious point, but one often lost in current policy discussions about how to attract and sustain a long-term care workforce. Understanding that there are both material and nonmaterial rewards associated with paid care work would, I suggest, move ongoing discussions about worker recruitment and retention beyond a limited focus on wages.

The caring self does raise a set of unanswered questions about the ability of workers to advocate for themselves collectively. Given that most aides in this study emphasize the intrinsic rewards of caregiving, such as cultivating companionship with clients, mobilizing for better wages and work conditions is not without its difficulties. In the next chapter, I consider the unionization of home care aides in both California and Ohio, paying particular attention to whether the caring self fosters or interferes with workers' mobilization.

4

ORGANIZING HOME CARE

MIKE, THE UNION ORGANIZER

On a late-summer evening in 2003, approximately twenty-five
home care aides gathered in a large meeting room of the IHSS main office
in Central City, California. The aides, new to IHSS but not necessarily to
home care, were there to attend a mandatory orientation session sponsored by the Public Authority for the county. The Public Authority is responsible for processing the wages of nearly ten thousand aides in Central
City and maintaining a registry that helps match workers with clients; it
serves as the official employer of record with whom aides may collectively
bargain. The orientation sessions, run by Public Authority social workers, provide aides with an introduction to the policies and procedures of
IHSS and help orient workers to their new jobs as quasi-public employees.
Since most of the aides who attend these workshops are hired directly by
a client, they are often surprised to learn that they will be paid through
the state, or IHSS (under the consumer-directed model, clients retain the

right to hire and fire, even though they do not directly pay workers). Orientation sessions also provide aides with their first exposure to the Service Employees International Union (SEIU), the union that represents home care aides in Central City. As I learned during the orientation session in 2003 and then in subsequent interviews and observations, aides possess conflicting views about the unionization of workers in their field. While some view unionization as an important step toward better wages and work conditions, others are vocal in their rejection of SEIU and of unionization more generally.

During this particular orientation, the social worker in charge began the session by offering the floor to Mike, a chief organizer for the local. Mike introduced himself as a longtime union man who had helped organize aides in institutional settings throughout California and was "in the trenches" in the years leading up to the significant union victory for home care workers in Los Angeles in 1999.[1] Aides in the room seemed either unimpressed or uninterested in Mike's organizing history, and others appeared downright hostile to his presence, rolling their eyes, muttering under their breath, and talking loudly over his voice. Mike explained that aides had recently voted for representation in Central City, after a nine-year battle with the county. The first contract was signed in 2001, guaranteeing workers a wage of $9.50 an hour and health care benefits to those working eighty-five hours or more per month. Mike reminded the aides in the room that these gains constituted significant improvements from the minimum wage a few years prior. The aides in the room, a diverse mix of Latinos, whites, African Americans, Asian Americans, and Russian Americans, appeared unmoved by Mike's summary of union perks. The tenor of the exchange changed notably, however, when Mike began to explain union dues.

Mike made clear that since all workers in Central City were represented by SEIU, there was a "fair share" policy in place that deducted 2 percent from gross wages each pay period for union dues. Handing around union membership cards as he spoke, Mike reiterated that while members are never obligated to sign union cards, dues are taken out of the wages of all IHSS aides since the union provides representation to all. Mike then launched into a plea for union volunteers, only to be cut off by a white woman in her midforties who was visibly unsettled. Identifying herself as someone who had worked for various home care agencies for nearly ten years, Mary Ann stood up and addressed the group about what she viewed as the "problem" of union dues. So angry she could barely construct a sentence, Mary Ann protested, "We are only making $7.50 an hour when you take out our dues!" Mike, un-shaken, explained that only 2 percent of gross would be deducted, for a maximum of twenty-two dollars per period, not two dollars an hour as Mary Ann believed. Further angered by his reply, Mary Ann raised her voice even louder, shouting, "You present yourself as a good program, but I'd like to see better presentation of what the union can offer us!"

Before Mike could respond, an African American woman who called herself Joanie stood up to defend the union. As someone who had worked for IHSS earlier in her life, she remembered a time when she re-ceived $4.25 an hour and was routinely undercompensated for her work. Without equivocation, Joanie concluded, "I would rather go for the union!" For nearly half an hour, Mike and the IHSS social worker allowed aides in the room to express their opinions on the subject of unions and union dues, a topic that sparked more interest among attendees than the discussion of payroll, criminal background checks, or training. The room appeared roughly split between those who possessed a clear dis-dain for unions generally and those who recognized the value, somewhat cautiously, of union representation. One woman in favor of the union commented quietly, "I am glad I am with a union because of health in-surance." To this, a young Asian American man replied, "Yes, but when are we going to get a 401(k) and paid leave?" This comment triggered a long discussion about the need for dental and vision coverage, some-thing the union had not yet secured. Mike reassured the group that the union would work for dental and vision coverage, but noted that unions are only as strong as their rank and file. And with that, Mike made one last plea for aides to sign their union cards. Seemingly inflamed by this last set of comments, Mary Ann interrupted one last time and offered her final thought for the day: "I thought I was American; I thought I have the right to choose [to be in a union]!" Sensing another digression com-ing, the social worker in charge of the orientation suggested that Mike leave the room so the group could turn to other topics.

Of the handful of Public Authority orientations I attended between 2001 and 2003, few erupted into such rancor over union representation. It was common, however, to witness open discussion about the value of unions, usually prompted by the realization that the local was "fair share" with respect to union dues. It became apparent that aides' beliefs and opinions about the union were shaped more by broad impressions of unions—often abstract and caricatured—rather than any concrete understanding of what unions do and why unions matter for workers, aides in particular. Moreover, nearly all of the aides I interviewed in both California and Ohio, with the exception of a few activists, were unaware of recent union victories in California and other states. Most expressed ambivalence or skepticism about the benefits of organizing, even when I talked with them about successful campaigns right in their backyards. Given the sizable organizing victory of SEIU in California in 1999, it surprised me that some of the aides in Central City did not believe that unionization was possible.

In this chapter, I describe aides' views on unions and unionization, offered to me by home care workers in both California and Ohio. Roughly half of the aides in both sites had something to say about unions, while the other half said they either knew too little to comment or didn't have much to say on the topic. Although I sample here from a small number of aides, their subjective views are nonetheless worthy of consideration. Much of the existing work on the unionization of home care workers summarizes organizing victories since the late nineties from either a historical or labor policy perspective (Boris and Klein 2006; Mareschal 2006, 2007). Although some of this work draws anecdotally on the experiences of aides heavily involved in union campaigns, the views of aides working in non-unionized states like Ohio are missing from these analyses, as are the perspectives of average rank-and-file workers in California and elsewhere. As Dan Clawson (2003) notes, "The most serious limitation of the new labor movement... is the failure to empower or activate the rank and file." Given this, I attempt to add the voices of rank-and-file home care workers to the existing scholarship on the unionization of careworkers, while also considering the perspectives of those workers not yet unionized.

It is important to note that data for this study were collected prior to controversies in 2008–9 in California involving SEIU leadership, namely, the misappropriation of funds by Local 6434 president, Tyrone Freeman, in Los Angeles, and the ongoing battle that started in 2009 in Northern California between the National Union of Healthcare Workers (a break-away union) and SEIU national leadership.[2] Although some aides express a degree of hesitancy about unions, their reluctance does not appear linked to controversies plaguing organized labor. Rather, aides' apprehension about unionization, in both California and Ohio, reflects a general lack of experience with and exposure to organized labor. This is not surprising, considering that union density is relatively low in the United States (about 13 percent) and that home care aides in particular are difficult to "reach" since there is no obvious shop floor or workplace culture. Even those aides represented by a union are ambivalent or unclear about the purpose of organized labor, since caregivers generally have very little contact with one another, let alone with the unions that represent them.

To help contextualize aides' accounts of unionization, I provide a brief summary of the status of union efforts in California and Ohio, paying particular attention to the notable labor victories for aides in the former. The beliefs and opinions about unions found among workers are then added to the discussion in an attempt address the aforementioned gap in the literature on home care unionization. I offer some conjecture as to whether—from the viewpoint of aides themselves—the relational and emotional nature of home care work, particularly bonds of companionship formed with clients, are incompatible with unionization. In other words, does the caring self impede or enable aides' beliefs in their collective rights as workers? This question is particularly important to consider in states like Ohio, where organizing efforts are nascent.

Organizing Home Care Workers in California and Ohio

California

In 1999, SEIU secured the largest union victory for organized labor since workers at Ford's River Rouge plant joined the United Auto Workers in 1941 (Delp and Quan 2002). After a nearly decade-long battle with the state of California over the rights of home care aides to collectively bargain, seventy-four thousand aides in Los Angeles County elected to join SEIU Local 434B. This significant triumph for labor symbolized a changing climate for home care workers in California, ushering in higher wages (now above ten dollars an hour in some counties), health care and dental benefits, and increased access to training (Howes 2005). These new conditions of work represented a marked improvement from the minimum wage previously earned by aides in California from the mid-1970s to the late 1990s. Union victories in New York, Washington, and Oregon occurred nearly simultaneously, improving conditions for aides living in those states as well (Mareschal 2006). While SEIU played (and continues to play) a principal role in organizing home care workers in California and elsewhere, other unions were also instrumental, including United Domestic Workers (UDW) and the American Federation of State, County, and Municipal Employees (AFSCME) (Mareschal 2006, 2007). Recently, unions like the National Union of Healthcare Workers (NUHW) have emerged as rivals to SEIU's dominance, especially in states like California.

During the California campaign of the late 1990's, aides working for IHSS were targeted by UDW as well as SEIU. IHSS was created in 1973 as part of the California Department of Social Services, charged with the task of administering publicly funded long-term care for poor elderly and disabled people. The roughly 441,000 aides in this system are quasi–public sector employees who provide care to 376,308 clients, or "consumers," in the state (California Association of Public Authorities for IHSS 2010). Roughly 40 percent of these aides are family providers, paid a wage by the state to care for their own relatives (Berg and Farrar 2000). Although clients are responsible for hiring and firing aides, pay is issued by the state-run IHSS program. The program is administered at the county level, with some counties supporting an "independent provider" model of care (where clients select their own caregivers) and others contracting care out to private or nonprofit agencies who manage care for the county (and for clients). In both contexts, unions encountered a significant hurdle on the road to organizing aides: Who was the employer with whom the union could bargain? Was it the state, the contracting private agencies, or elderly and disabled clients?

Not surprisingly, the California Department of Social Services resisted being codified as the employer of record, insisting that clients played that role. After a series of unsuccessful lawsuits filed by SEIU to try to position the state as employer, the union led a coalition of consumer groups in an effort to change the law at the level of the state legislature. Ultimately, the union helped usher through the Public Authorities Act of 1992, which permitted counties to create public authorities to serve as employer of record. Aides did not become county employees under this arrangement, remaining "independent providers" who could still be hired and fired by consumers (Mareschal 2006). Importantly, though, public authorities established a way for aides to bargain collectively for higher wages and benefits, although intense effort was required on the part of SEIU and UDW to lobby each county to establish an authority. Some counties were receptive to the idea, while others—like Los Angeles—presented significant challenges (Delp and Quan 2002; Mareschal 2006). As of 2009, California had fifty-six public authorities, out of a total of fifty-eight counties, with whom workers bargain directly.

Several factors contributed to the successful campaign in California, including a crucial alliance between home care aides and consumers, specifically a coalition between SEIU, Centers for Independent Living, the World Institute on Disability, and the California Senior Legislature (Delp and Quan 2002; Mareschal 2006). While this was not a seamless alliance (Boris and Klein 2006), a display of unity between consumer and provider groups helped sustain the frame that client care, not simply worker wages, was at stake. As such, the unions engaged in a form of "symbolic management" (Ashforth and Gibbs, in Mareschal 2006, 42) that promoted worker interests as deeply aligned with those of the dependent elderly and disabled.

Unionization certainly improved the working conditions of home care workers in California, with some variation by county. Wages rose to over nine dollars an hour, and aides working over a certain number of hours per month—determined by each county—became eligible for health benefits. Improvements in wages and benefits have been linked to improvements statewide in worker recruitment and retention (Howes 2005, 2006). In addition, public authorities now offer ongoing training sessions for workers, including seminars about how to properly "transfer" (lift) clients, how to implement universal precautions in the workplace, and how to manage the emotional toll of caregiving. The authorities also administer background checks on providers at the request and expense of consumers, while also maintaining a registry of aides to ensure that clients and caregivers are easily matched.

SEIU and other unions also provide aides some degree of protection when the state decides to trim money from the publicly supported IHSS program. Funding for the public authorities was not written into the initial 1992 legislation; financial support later came from Medicaid dollars, with the state and the counties splitting the remaining obligation (Mareschal 2006). This arrangement leaves IHSS—including workers and clients—vulnerable to cuts when state budget crises emerge. In 2004, Governor Schwarzenegger proposed major cuts to the IHSS program, backing off only after consumers pressured his administration to secure additional federal funds to offset the deficit (Mareschal 2006). During the budget crisis of 2009, the legislature passed a budget plan trimming the IHSS program by $226 million, citing concerns about rampant fraud in the system. As part of the proposed cuts, Schwarzenegger also pushed through mandatory fingerprinting of both clients and consumers. Although the decrease in funding and increased surveillance constitutes a significant blow to the IHSS program, SEIU did manage to block—through court injunction—the state's attempt to lower the hourly wage of workers from $12.10 to $10.70 (inclusive of benefits). So while the union cannot prevent massive social service spending cuts at the state level, which indirectly affect both clients and consumers, they do have some power to prevent California from balancing the budget by slashing the wages of low-wage home care aides.

A significant drawback of the public authority model is that it generally does not provide collective bargaining rights to aides working for private, for-profit home care companies. Among aides in this study, the workers employed by It's For You, for example, were not unionized, knew very little about the possibility of a union, and had lower hourly wages and fewer benefits than IHSS workers. Additionally, under the public authority system, workers bargain directly with counties, so there is a great deal of variation in the wages and benefits offered workers throughout the state. In places like Sacramento, San Francisco, and Los Angeles, wages are relatively high (over nine dollars per hour), whereas some rural counties continue to pay aides minimum wage and offer few or no benefits. Thus, the public authority model indirectly reinforces disparities across the state with respect to fair compensation (Mareschal 2006).

Even so, the California story is an important success in terms of the sheer number of aides unionized, as well as the creative way in which an employer of record, via the public authority system, was established. As Mareschal (2006) notes, however, victories in states like California, Oregon, and elsewhere were products of innovation and adaptation on the part of unions who had to navigate the complicated quasi-public nature of home care services. Accordingly, she cautions the labor movement from "blindly emulating" the California model and suggests that organizers instead pay close attention to the "political environments and opportunity structures" that vary by state (26). This is especially true in states like Ohio, where the movement to organize home care workers is in its infancy. Given the recent controversies surrounding SEIU, including infighting with other service unions, it remains to be seen whether California's labor victories will be replicated in states like Ohio.

Ohio

The story of unionization in Ohio is necessarily a much shorter tale, since the campaign to organize aides in the state began relatively recently. In 2007, Governor Strickland signed Executive Order 23S, which granted collective bargaining rights to independent home health care workers in the state. These "independent contractors" provide Medicaid-reimbursed direct care services that are administered by various social service agencies at the state level, such as the Department of Aging, Job and Family Services, and Mental Retardation. In justifying his actions, Strickland cited the need to improve long-term care services in the state as the primary motivator for extending bargaining rights to home care aides, while also making the point that the right to organize has already been granted to aides working in nursing homes. Although the executive order was heralded as an important step forward by labor advocates in Ohio, it remains unclear exactly how many aides will benefit from the governor's directive.

Like IHSS workers in California, aides covered under the executive order are paid a wage by the state to care for a low-income elderly or disabled person (sometimes a relative), as part of Ohio's Medicaid waiver program. Even though aides in Ohio are paid by the government and their jobs administered by government agencies, independent contractors are not considered to be public or state employees. In fact, on a government website that provides information on the state home care program, prospective providers are encouraged to think of themselves as entrepreneurs starting a new business. Ohio home care workers, then, face a challenge similar the one that confronted IHSS aides in California: establishing an employer of record with whom to bargain.[3]

Early in fall 2007, only months after Strickland signed his order, SEIU 1199 secured the right to represent seven thousand independent providers. In 2008, the union voted on their first contract, increasing wages and benefits for SEIU home care workers employed through the Medicaid waiver program. It is important to note that roughly two thousand of the seven thousand independent providers organized by SEIU are skilled home health nurses, not home care aides. While reliable estimates of the total population of home care aides in Ohio are not available, the BLS reports that in 2009 there were 13,010 personal and home care aides in the state (Bureau of Labor Statistics 2009). These numbers suggest that while the unionization of independent providers is a significant symbolic victory, the majority of aides in the state are not represented. Furthermore, Strickland's executive order specifically precludes representation for aides employed by private agencies, leaving these workers with little recourse when it comes to unfair wages and benefits. As the story in Ohio unfolds, SEIU and other unions will likely have to adapt to the complex terrain of public and private home care services in Ohio, just as they have done in states like California, New York, Oregon, and Washington.[4]

Workers' Perspectives on Unions

Since the primary goal of this study is to understand the nature of home care from the perspective of aides, particularly how they experience and manage the emotional labor of paid caregiving, questions about unions remained tangential to the research. Although I did interview aides in California for whom organizing was a high priority,[5] aides generally did not bring up the topic of unionization. When the subject was raised during a training, a gathering, or an interview, aides had relatively little positive or negative to say about unions. This is perhaps somewhat of an obvious finding, since rates of unionization are low in the United States relative to other Western industrial nations (Voss and Sherman 2000) and worker attitudes toward unions are reluctant at best and hostile at worst (Clawson 2003; Lopez 2004; Voss and Sherman 2000). Even so, aides—especially in the Rust Belt city of Middletown—did talk about what they view as the pros and cons of unionization and what they see as the primary impediments or challenges to collective bargaining.

Ohio

When I interviewed agency-based home care aides, all women, in Middletown, Ohio, in 2008, the governor of the state had passed the executive order the year before that granted collective bargaining rights to independent home care aides (those not employed by the state or by private agencies). More recently, these independent providers—constituting roughly seven thousand of the one hundred thirty thousand aides in Ohio—elected to be represented by SEIU 1199. Aides interviewed in Middletown all worked for a private agency and were not unionized. None of the aides were aware that SEIU had organized independent providers in the state, and only one aide had heard of unionizing victories in other states such as California and New York. Even though the women seemed "out of the loop" with respect to unionization, most had tempered, albeit cautious, views on the matter.

Tammy, of Middletown, responds this way when I ask her about the possibility of unionizing home care workers in Ohio:

> I don't think it's a yes-or-no question. I've been a union advocate for many, many years and was involved in trying to organize at Central State University at one point in the 1980s. First of all, I want to say, you have to be so careful about the union that you bring in. I can think of one, right now, that I would consider unionizing health care workers. But I'm out of that loop; I really don't know exactly what's out there. You know, for a while, they were called Nine to Five. They are the Communications Workers of America. Just as I said that, I know there's another, but I can't remember the name of that union.

She goes on to say that unions might prove especially useful when it comes to training and protecting workers who take on the inherent risks of caring for an elderly or disabled person in the home. Tammy believes that training aides to manage the risks of the job is as important as improving wages and benefits, commenting that "somebody really needs to take hold of the industry, all these agencies, and do some kind of regulation. Increase the criteria for home care aides." For Tammy, proper training is tied directly to the quality of care that she and her peers can provide clients. In her view, unions can push for much-needed change with respect to training:

> In a situation where, if you're with a client, you're not allowed to perform CPR, but you know it has to be done, most people are going to do it. They're going to take the risk. You're going to weigh the risk against the benefits. If you get fired, you get fired. But I do think if we have an organization behind this that provided training, like a union, that would also address benefits, then we could do a lot better job.

While she views unionization as overwhelmingly positive, Tammy is skeptical that agencies would welcome organized labor, namely because of the potential loss of revenue:

> Health care agencies, frankly, like it the way it is. They really can hire people off the street. And they get lucky a lot of times. Sometimes they don't. But once somebody gets behind this industry and starts demanding training and actually comes up with a manual, it's not going to be so easy for these agencies anymore. The pay is going to go up. It'll have to go up. The training is just going to be—it'll be very expensive. And agencies are very profitable and one of the reasons is because they don't have to... worry about us as a profession.

Tammy is correct to assume that private agencies resist unionization, although there certainly have been successful organizing campaigns in states where agencies predominate (Mareschal 2006). Many agencies subcontract with the state for Medicaid and Medicare dollars, which means that few private agencies operate in a truly independent way. In some states, such as New York, agencies' dependency on federal and state reimbursements has translated into leverage for workers, since agencies rely on the support of organized labor when lobbying for increased spending on home care (Mareschal 2006). In exchange for this support from unions, agencies concede to higher wages and benefits for workers. Aides like Tammy, however, are generally unaware of such possibilities and remain skeptical about unionization in Ohio.

Beyond the issue of organizing, Tammy wonders whether it is even possible to translate what she does into a "fair wage." When I ask her to elaborate, she speaks about the unquantifiable value of the care she and others provide. Her colleague Lucy comes to mind, an aide who has worked for nearly forty years as a paid caregiver, taking on "difficult clients" with enthusiasm. Tammy is unsure whether raising her friend's wages a few dollars would serve as adequate compensation:

> I know an aide who has very difficult clients. She works more than forty hours a week. Her job is very physical and unpleasant. And when I think of what I do, and I think about what I should be making, it's hard for me to think in those terms. The aide [Lucy] that I have met who's told me the intensity of her job, she should be making fifty thousand dollars a year. She's

everything to these people. You know, she's counseling, she's a sounding board, she just does everything....I wonder if she could be paid enough for what she does. You know?

For another aide, Maggie, the fact that aides are so central to the well-being of clients is precisely the reason why compensation and benefits should improve. She believes that "they need to give aides recognition because aides are with people. They're working six to eight to ten to twelve hours a day. They know what's going on more than the family could ever think of knowing." Maggie views unionization in a positive light, and thinks that "they [aides] do need something formed" if for no other reason than to remind caregivers that they have value. She believes that if aides were to receive such recognition in the form of higher wages, there would be considerably less turnover. Even though she is overwhelmingly in support of a union, Maggie doubts it is possible, citing lack of contact between aides:

> In agencies you don't have contact with other aides. They should have a meeting at least once a month, really, where other aides get to know other aides, to talk about clients. Communication is the key to everything. It's not good [in agencies]. There's nothing...just no communicating.

Maggie astutely identifies one of the key impediments to unionizing home care aides: there is no "shop floor" where workers congregate and develop solidarity, making it difficult for organizers to track down and unite workers (Delp and Quan 2002). Home care victories in California and other states have been achieved largely through a combination of neighborhood and grassroots organizing, legislative and political tactics, and coalition building with advocacy groups like Gray Panthers or activists in the independent living movement (Boris and Klein 2006; Delp and Quan 2002; Mareschal 2006, 2007). There is little doubt that SEIU intends to use similar tactics in states like Ohio, likely with some degree of success, but it is nonetheless difficult for aides "in the trenches" of caregiving to imagine unionization in real terms, given how isolated they are from one another.

Virginia, sixty-two, is overwhelmingly positive about a union, more for the benefit of younger workers than herself. She identifies herself as "on the way out" of the occupation and doesn't believe that unionization will be achieved before she retires. Virginia hopes, though, that unionization

will improve conditions for the working mothers who are trying to provide for children on a meager wage. She explains:

> So if this is a possibility,...if somebody can do something with the union,
> I think that would be awesome. I'm going to get Social Security here pretty
> soon, and it isn't going to be a heck of a lot, so I'm still going to have to work.
> But I'm on my way out. You know that. I don't know how much longer I'll
> be able to do it. But the aides that are out there...I mean, God bless these
> women who come in and—maybe they're getting a divorce so they're in
> charge of the family. If they love what they're doing, and a lot of them do,
> you know, they really care about this type of thing, I would fight for their
> right to be able to go on and do that [form a union]. Absolutely. The need is
> there. They're not using LPNs like they used to. And the RNs don't want to
> get their hands dirty. I mean, who do you think cleans up the poop and does
> all of that, you know?...I really think there ought to be some kind of pro-
> gram. And it's long overdue. I wish I could have had it for my time.

Dot, for her part, is keenly aware of the injustices of being a home care
provider, so much so that she has considered taking a job at Walmart.
When asked what she thinks of unionizing as one way to achieve higher
wages and better benefits, her initial reaction is, "I've never even thought
about it. And I'm not sure how they, to be honest with you, how you really
could do it." To this, Dot adds, "I'm not really sure how much unions help
anymore. I think a lot of people think that." The idea of paying dues to
an ineffectual union is also unpalatable to Dot, who clearly has conflicting
views about whether caregiving should be the subject of collective bargaining. For example, Dot talks at length about taking a pay cut to remain with
one of her clients, who switched to an agency that offered aides two dollars less an hour. When I suggest that unionization might standardize pay
across agencies, at least ideally, she responds that "money is not the reason
I do this job."

Like many other U.S. workers, and other aides interviewed, Dot is
dismayed by "do-nothing unionism" (Lopez 2004) and is not convinced
that unions in their current form can improve the lives of aides. Living in the Rust Belt city of Middletown, Dot has probably experienced
job loss directly or indirectly, and is aware of the weakened power of
unions in a rapidly deindustrializing region of the United States. In such
a context, it is not surprising that Dot needs to be convinced of the value

of (or even the existence of) a service union. Additionally, Dot—like many other aides—proudly narrates her caring self, declaring that she is not in care work for the money. While this presentation of the caring self allows Dot to reaffirm an altruistic commitment to her clients, she struggles to find language to talk about care as work and her need for fair compensation.

California

Aides working in Central City, California, share with workers in Ohio many of the same cautiously optimistic views about unionization. The caregivers in Central City are a more diverse group, by race, ethnicity, and gender, but it is difficult, given the sample size, to attribute any variation in views about unionization to differences of social location. It is worth noting, however, that views on unionization tend to be more extreme among California aides, with workers either vociferously supporting SEIU's efforts or wholly rejecting organized labor. Even though IHSS workers in Central City were unionized nearly two years prior to this study, most aides knew few details about the union and a small number of IHSS workers were unaware that SEIU represented them. Sandra, for example, a caregiver working for a private agency, voiced strong opposition to a union "coming in," unaware that SEIU had already organized IHSS workers in the city:

> I would not be a CNA if they brought a union in. I will not work for a union. I worked for the Teamsters. Need I say more? I will not work for a union ever again. I mean, they say one thing and do something else, you know? They can't be trusted. As far as I'm concerned, they just can't be trusted.

Like Sandra, several aides had previous experiences with unions that soured them to the idea of representation. Camilla, an aide working for the same private agency as Sandra, had been represented by a service union while employed as an aide in a facility for the mentally ill. During a night shift, Camilla was stabbed with a pencil by a resident, a wound that required a visit to the emergency room and extensive stitches to her arm. After the incident, Camilla was fired without explanation. Seeking counsel from the union, Camilla learned that they couldn't help her because she was not employed full-time, a technicality that angered her:

> Now my only thing about the union is...I had dealt with them when I lost my job at the facility. They don't help you. They don't really ask to help you, you know. And then they [the union] told me, if I would have been full-time,...they [the employer] couldn't have done nothing to me. But by me being on call and part-time, they [the union] couldn't do nothing. But I'm paying you dues every month....Come on!

Michael, an IHSS aide in Central City, has mixed feelings about unions. On the one hand, he believes that home care workers need help from "somebody" since their caregiving commitments prevent them from pulling out of jobs where the working conditions are poor. As he put it, "You can't walk away." When I ask if SEIU provides any of the protections and benefits he is looking for, Michael seems unsure. He claims to have "sort of supported" the aides advocating for a union in the late 1990s, but adds that he didn't really understand the purpose of all the effort. Worrying that the union is too "political," Michael chooses not to get involved: "I felt compelled, but I didn't really want to do that much because I didn't really know what was going on. I don't want to do something that I don't know about, you know? If I don't believe in it, I won't do it. It's just hypocrisy."

Several aides echo Michael's concerns about not understanding the purpose of the union or not knowing enough to get involved, although most concede that the wage and benefit protections secured by SEIU are significant. Three aides working for IHSS have strong opinions in favor of the union. One woman, Karen, worked for the union in the hope of professionalizing the work and improving the quality of care:

> You can't just go in there and wash the dishes, throw some food in, and take off. If you are paying them minimum wage, that's what you're going to get. That's all you're paying for. That's why I am working with the union and the Public Authority: to, first of all, make a profession that's worth being a profession.

Andrew, an aide employed by IHSS as well as a private agency, agrees with Karen that quality of care is tied to higher wages. Additionally, he sees unionization as one way that aides can more readily dedicate themselves to clients. For Andrew, union representation and higher wages must be present for aides to enact their caring selves. He explains:

> I think it's important [the union]. They've opened up a lot of doors for in-home support care work. I just could never believe that the average home care worker would be making $9.50 an hour. Just a few years ago they were making about $4.25 or $5.50. With the cost of living like it is and the type of work—And you had to pay for your own gas and have transportation to get to these people. Some of these people [clients] want to remain being independent and living on their own, and the only way that can happen is if they have someone come in there and assist them with health care. Someone that they can trust; someone that's honest, sincere, and dedicated. So when the pay rate goes up, that changes things for people, makes it where they can dedicate themselves.... You know, I can pay my bills a little bit better now. I can't pay my bills at $4.25 or $5.50 an hour. I got kids and stuff like that, so I have to work two or three other jobs, so it means it cuts them down to a point of what kind of quality they can give that person.

Joyce, an aide working for IHSS, sees unionization less from the perspective of client care and more from the vantage point of the frustrated worker. She is thankful that there is an outlet for workers who feel aggrieved. Joyce concedes that unions can't always resolve disputes in the workplace, but believes there is some value in simply having a "place to go": "Being in a union is fine. It gives you someplace to go and scream and holler, you know? Somebody you can gripe and complain to. You won't always get things done, but you have somebody you can verbally express your feelings to."

Given significant union victories for home care workers in California, it was surprising to encounter only a handful of aides who, like Joyce, explicitly support the union. Although these findings can in no way claim to be representative of the larger population of home care workers in Northern California, the ambivalence and opposition to unions voiced by aides hint at the challenges organizers face when activating rank and file. This may be especially true for aides currently working in California, where infighting and jurisdictional battles between unions for membership have received considerable attention in the press.

So many of the aides working in home care live below or just above the poverty line, often juggling multiple clients and sometimes multiple jobs to make ends meet. It should come as little surprise, then, that aides are often oblivious to unionization campaigns and underwhelmed at the thought of becoming active members. Take, for example, Mark, an aide living in Central City, who estimates that he bikes thirty miles a day in order to reach his various clients in the suburbs of Central City (occasionally sleeping in bus stops overnight to ensure he is close and available to a client living a good distance from his apartment). How could Mark possibly fit union organizing into his life? How would he even hear about the union? How might a union organizer find him to persuade him of the benefits of representation and becoming active?

It is also clear from the accounts above that many workers have prior, albeit limited, experiences with unions, experiences that have negatively colored their view of labor. Overcoming perceptions that unions "do nothing" for workers is a difficult challenge for SEIU and others who seek to organize home care aides. Even in places where unions have achieved success, activating the rank and file will depend on the ability of organizers to make clear that "new labor" has something to offer service workers, aides in particular. If the opinions of aides related here are any indication, cynicism about the power of unions is deeply entrenched in the collective psyche of workers. So much so that promises of higher wages and better benefits are not enough to convince aides that a union is worthwhile. Without a compelling frame for why aides should accept and join a union, most appear ambivalent, while others resent what they see as yet another bureaucratic intrusion into their lives. Perhaps it is unrealistic to expect organized labor to reinvent itself, and make itself attractive to more workers, when there is currently little agreement across sectors of the labor movement itself about how to move forward and improve union density.[6] Even so, making a compelling case about how unions have changed and why they are important for workers—all workers—may help labor sway home care aides to unionize or, if already organized, to participate in an existing union.

The silver lining in this story is that aides generally do not view caring commitments as incompatible with self-advocacy in the workplace. Some, like Dot, struggle to articulate how much care work is "worth," at the same time making clear that wages and conditions of work are unfavorable. Much more commonly, aides argue that higher wages and better benefits are a *necessary* part of providing quality care and ensuring "dedication" to clients. For these aides, having a good job with fair compensation is conducive to, not a detraction from, their caring selves. Successful union campaigns in California, Oregon, and New York are keenly aware of this connection aides feel between their own work conditions and client quality of care (Boris and Klein 2006; Delp and Quan 2002; Mareschal 2007). As such, organizing to date has been framed around the needs of both workers and clients, so that any agitation for improved working conditions is seen as a way to improve services for the elderly and disabled, rather than a ploy for higher wages by "greedy" workers (Mareschal 2006).

Future campaigns will be wise to follow in the footsteps of service unions that place the caregiver-client *relationship* at the center of organizing efforts. Doing so will ensure that workers, especially inactive rank and file, more readily relate to union efforts; will help foster and sustain existing alliances between home care workers, citizen groups, and social movement organizations (such as the independent living movement); and will make worker demands more palatable to the general public. Remaining focused on the relational nature of home care work might also help organizers "win over" workers—aides not yet organized, as well as existing rank and file—who, some for good reason, harbor a deep distrust of unions. In short, the caring selves of workers should be taken seriously by organizers, not just as an abstract identity formation, but as a movement resource that, if activated wisely, will enhance ongoing campaigns for unionization.

Conclusion

Improving the Conditions of Paid Caregiving

Sooner or later, most of us will confront the limitations of our system of long-term care firsthand, as we face illness or disability in our own lives or the lives of loved ones. For a very few, ample personal resources will mean high-quality care, in the comfort of a home or reputable facility, provided by a team of professional and paraprofessional caregivers. For another subset—the very poor—services will be pieced together with the help of family, friends, and the state. For the vast majority of us, there will be a series of tough decisions to make about the location of care (home or facility), how care will be paid for, and who will provide the care. In the current context, such decisions are agonizing and, often, result in less-than-desirable outcomes, like "spending down" one's assets before receiving state support, placing a loved one in substandard care, or leaving a job because of caring commitments to family.

Much has been made of the inadequate patchwork of medical and social services that make up long-term care in the United States. With great alarm, scholars and policymakers draw our attention to the "care gap" or "care crisis" facing U.S. families, noting the anticipated growth in the number of dependent elderly and the insufficient number of caregivers available to care for them (Institute of Medicine of the National Academies 2008). Additionally, there is a great deal of concern about the quality of care provided to the elderly and disabled, in both home and institutional contexts. Families subsequently worry, for good reason, whether they can entrust facilities and providers with the care of a loved one. In sum, the availability and quality of long-term care services appear to be of paramount importance to families and consumers of care.

Generally missing from this public conversation about long-term care are frontline workers like nursing aides. These are the women and men who staff nursing facilities; who travel daily to care for clients in the home; and who provide the bulk of companionship services and custodial care to the disabled, mentally ill, and elderly in our communities. If the elderly are invisible and disenfranchised, as some have argued (Calasanti and Slevin 2001), then the aides who care for them are even more hidden from public interest and attention. And yet without these frontline workers, bodies would not be washed, dressed, or exercised; medications would likely go unadministered; and many elderly and disabled people would spend much of their time completely alone. Aides working in nursing facilities or private homes do much of the "dirty work" that families can't or won't do, and that doctors and nurses provide at higher costs to consumers, if they provide it at all. In short, direct care workers are the backbone and driving force of long-term care in the United States.

This book attempts to enrich our understanding of long-term care from the perspective of aides themselves, bringing to light both the inequalities and rewards associated with the work. The honest and sometimes moving accounts offered by the women and men of Central City and Middletown humanize a population of workers who are generally ignored and sometimes stigmatized by public figures and the press. While fraud and negligence are no doubt part of home care, just as they are part of any medical or social service, home care workers appear to be—and certainly feel—stigmatized by a broader public that does not understand what they do.

By listening to what paid caregivers have to say about what attracts them to the work, what keeps them in the job, and what prompts them to leave, we not only improve our understanding of aides as professionals but also begin to chip away at the problem of burnout and turnover in the field. While there is a great deal already written on the rates and causes of turnover among aides in nursing homes, very little research explores work constraints facing home care workers specifically (Brannon et al. 2002; Ejaz et al. 2008; Seavey 2004). There is strong evidence that poor pay and lack of benefits contribute to turnover and burnout among home-based workers, and that increased compensation improves retention (Howes 2005, 2006, 2008). Judging by the accounts collected in this book, however, the emotional conditions of work, in addition to the material, are also central to workers' sense of job satisfaction and identity. I suggest these relational aspects of the job are just as important as monetary compensation, for it is through connections to clients that aides construct a workplace identity—the caring self—and achieve a sense of dignity at work. This is not to say that aides remain caregivers solely for the emotional rewards, but rather that both material and nonmaterial factors play an important role in their job satisfaction. If we are to truly understand the complex problems of turnover and burnout, we must take seriously the emotional dimensions of paid care work and systematically examine the role that emotions play in producing both positive and negative work experiences.

A closer look at home care aides, for example, reveals that the relational nature of paid caregiving compels aides to withstand unfair work conditions or willingly offer uncompensated care to clients. Precisely because aides derive a great deal of personal value from their personal ties with clients, going "above and beyond" serves simultaneously to assert the caring self and to obscure a potentially exploitive work arrangement. Given this reality, the relational work of paid caregiving is a source of both *inequality* and *identity* for home care aides. As Uttal and Tuominen (1999) note, this tension between the exploitations and emotional rewards of care work is common in contexts such as home-based child care or elder care, where laborers form genuine attachments to their charges. This book offers a detailed account of one occupational group's experiences managing both the inequality and identity work associated with home-based labor.

Inequality in Home Care

While aides' emotional connections to clients are central to their job satisfaction and sense of self on the job, there are a number of inequalities associated with home care work. These constraints should be carefully considered by those shaping long-term care in the United States, especially policymakers seeking solutions to the staffing crisis. Specifically, low wages as well as lack of benefits such as health care and paid sick leave sustain inequality in paid caregiving, such that three in ten direct care workers live near or below the poverty line (Paraprofessional Healthcare Institute 2008a). It is a poor commentary on our long-term care system that we in the United States do not offer a living wage or health care to all caregivers who tend to our elderly and disabled on a daily basis.[1] Aides also experience inequality at the hands of agencies that provide poor support or supervision and implicitly condone a "don't ask, don't tell" approach to patient care. Home care workers are offered very little training by agencies, but are nonetheless asked by clients to perform specialized tasks such as cleaning necrotic tissue, removing a catheter, or injecting insulin. Formally forbidden from carrying out these tasks, aides still assume the risk because there are few others to provide care.

When agencies do step in to define aides' scope of work, it is in ways that sometimes seem at cross-purposes to client care. Some aides, for example, are forbidden from driving clients to appointments or taking them for a walk to the park due to liability concerns. Most are told to remain "professionally detached" from clients, to the point where they are given little time to grieve when a client passes away. As we learn from the caregivers in this book, however, emotional norms and feeling rules in home care are more suggestive of family than a formal employer-employee relationship. When agencies ignore this reality in the name of professionalism, they deny what is in fact central to both quality care and worker satisfaction: emotional ties to clients and their families.

Forming close connections to clients is not without its drawbacks, however. Emotional labor can also have harmful consequences for aides' well-being, especially over sustained periods of time. As predicted by the literature on emotional labor in service occupations, aides do describe a degree of alienation, frustration, and even boredom that can happen after months or years of engaging in emotion work with elderly and disabled clients. This reality, combined with low wages, confirms Macdonald and Sirianni's (1996) assertion that paid careworkers are the "emotional proletariat" of the service sector. Aides in this study report a certain degree of emotional overinvestment in clients that leads to burnout, while also testifying that they feel emotionally fatigued when dealing with negligent, absent, or overly directive families. Perhaps most troubling of all, many home care aides give care to clients *in surplus,* above and beyond what they are contracted to provide. Whether this amounts to staying a few hours after the formal end of a shift, answering phone calls from clients in the middle of the night, or offering their own money to clients, aides are often the ones clients turn to when they need additional care or support.

The problem of surplus care is particularly acute for home care workers, where the boundaries of family and work, and the feeling rules associated with those spaces, are considerably blurred. Since aides take seriously the task of cultivating companionship with clients, it sometimes becomes difficult for them to identify when and how to erect boundaries. Even though providing surplus care to elderly or disabled clients may "feel right" in the moment, most aides admit that, over time, overextending themselves for clients can lead to feelings of frustration or emotional exhaustion. The lesson here is that the emotional labor of home care is a source of alienation and fatigue, at the same time that it fosters job satisfaction and a positive sense of self on the job. Since providers' surplus care is also a likely source of burnout for aides, it makes sense that we begin thinking about ways to support and reward aides for their willingness to go "above and beyond" (through overtime compensation, for example). Aides also need training to help them understand how and when to erect clear emotional boundaries with clients. Given the tendency of home care aides to become fictive family, agencies must recognize the inevitability of aide-client companionship and then support workers accordingly. The first step, however, is recognizing and taking seriously the role of emotional labor in the work lives of aides.

The Rewards of Care: Autonomy, Dignity, and Identity

Aides in both Middletown and Central City are very clear about the rewards, emotional and otherwise, of working in home care. Many of the women and men in the field have years of experience working in institutions or assisted living facilities where constraints on care are profound. These aides welcome the change to home care, after losing tolerance for institutional work that compromises their autonomy and violates personal standards of care. Home care, by contrast, affords aides a higher degree of relational autonomy relative to institutional care, and fosters fictive kinship bonds between aides and their clients. The freedom to provide care as one sees fit, along with pseudofamilial ties to clients, sets the stage for the development of the caring self, an identity formation common to all aides interviewed. The caring self allows aides to minimize any stigma that comes from doing "dirty work," at the same time that it promotes paid caregiving as an altruistic service to others that only a select few are equipped to handle. Aides construct the caring self in a way that allows them to create a strong occupational culture and minimize the "occupational taint" associated with their low-skilled labor (Ashforth and Kreiner 1999; Ashforth et al. 2007; Drew, Mills, and Gassaway 2007).

Caring selves are narrated as natural or essential social identities that downplay the fact that home care is a form of waged labor. Aides emphasize their natural dispositions to care, rather than the "constrained choices" (Bird and Rieker 2008) that propel most of them into careers of unpaid and paid care work. This narrative of care leaves intact the caring self and reinforces the notion that aides are engaged in altruistically motivated, socially valuable work. While clearly identity-affirming, the essentialized and sometimes gendered language of the caring self can undermine aides' ability to employ a language of *labor* to talk about what they do, at least on an individual level. For example, most aides know they are underpaid, but very few are able to articulate what their care is worth in terms of a wage. Some argue that it is difficult to "put a price" on caregiving because of the emotional and relational tasks associated with the work.

The good news is that the caring self does not appear to preclude workers from *collectively* advocating for improved wages and benefits, as organizing campaigns in Oregon, California, and Washington attest. Unions seem well aware that successful organizing drives must, on some level, place clients (and aides' relationships to clients) at center, thereby validating the caring selves of workers. Reinforcing, as SEIU and other unions do, that better jobs equal better care for clients has proved a successful strategy of persuasion for service unions interested in organizing home care workers. Although there are lingering questions about the effectiveness of service unions in activating and communicating with existing rank and file (Clawson 2003), the recent story of home care unionization suggests that identity—that is, the caring self—does not reinforce workplace inequality.

If anything, playing to the caring self has been an important rhetorical strategy of unions seeking wage *equality* for home care workers.

The tension between inequality and identity, as presented throughout the book, is likely of interest to sociologists of work and occupations who seek to understand how workers subjectively manage and interpret their structurally disadvantaged positions within the labor market. By contrast, scholars and policymakers interested in long-term care may wonder how the preceding discussion relates to the "real world" problems of staffing, turnover, and burnout, all of which threaten the quality of long-term care in the United States. To address this, I first offer a hypothetical anecdote.

Imagine a scenario where an aide, Marty, a fifteen-year veteran of home care, regularly spends the night at the home of a very elderly client, Neera, even though she is discouraged from doing so by her agency and is uncompensated for the overnight hours. Marty has known her client for nearly five years and has watched the elderly woman's condition worsen and her social ties diminish. Likening their relationship to a mother-daughter bond, Marty provides surplus care to Neera because she is invested in her well-being and worries about her being left alone. After several months of caring for Neera and juggling her daytime clients, Marty grows fatigued and frustrated by the workload. She notices that the night shift is affecting the quality of care she provides other clients (she is impatient, unable to concentrate) and she is experiencing some secondary health problems from months of interrupted sleep. Unable to get out of bed one morning out of sheer exhaustion, Marty calls her agency and tells them that she would like to take some time off. Although sympathetic, the agency owner cannot offer Marty paid leave and so Marty quits. The following week, Marty travels to her sister's home in a nearby town where she finds a part-time job answering phones for a local business. Marty resolves to stay out of home care for a while, until she feels emotionally and physically able to do the work again.

Marty's story, though hypothetical, is a composite of the many stresses and strains affecting home care aides today. Given what we know about high rates of turnover and burnout, Marty's case might lead one to assume that she overinvested emotionally and physically in her client, experiencing burnout as a result of the psychosocial demands of caregiving. To be sure, Marty appears to have suffered emotionally and psychologically as a result of her intense commitment to Neera. But is emotional burnout the only potential source of strain in this scenario? What is the interplay between Marty's emotional labor and the structural context of her work?

Although feelings of emotional exhaustion were somewhat inevitable in Marty's case, I suggest that aides might experience the strain of their emotional output differently depending on the structural conditions of work, such as fair wages, adequate training, and options for paid and unpaid leave. It is not difficult to imagine an alternate outcome to Marty's situation, where she experiences the same degree of emotional strain but is able to manage the stress because she has options for respite; adequate professional training to handle the signs and symptoms of burnout; and fair compensation that allows her to focus on those caregiving assignments (like Neera) that matter most. As scholars and policymakers continue to study the link between emotional labor and burnout or turnover for low-skilled health workers, it is imperative that research consider the microinteractional, organizational, and macrostructural forces that have an impact on workers' emotional output. Doing so will turn attention away from our seemingly exclusive focus on individual level factors associated with burnout and turnover, toward the institutional and structural constraints that provide context for the interactional work of caregiving.

Making Home Care a Good Job

If direct care workers, specifically aides, are the backbone of long-term care in the United States, then efforts to make home care a good job should be of the highest priority. Fair compensation is perhaps the most obvious and critical step to ensuring a robust home care workforce. Unionization, as discussed in chapter 4, is critical to aides' efforts to secure better wages and benefits. In California, we know that unionization has significantly improved wages for home care aides and that, as a result, workers in that state are less likely to leave the job (Howes 2005, 2006). Organizing aides may also translate into improved access to training, as happened in California under the public authority system. On the heels of victories in Oregon, New York, Illinois, and Washington, service unions appear well poised to increase the number of aides represented by organized labor in the United States, provided that the labor movement can get beyond persistent problems of infighting and public scandal. The sticky problem of

how and whether aides employed by private agencies can be organized remains, although in certain states (like California) private agencies present less of a problem because of the sheer number of aides working for the
state as quasi–public sector employees.

Although organizing aides state by state promises to improve the wages
and working conditions of home care workers over time, there are other
changes at the federal level that must be considered. Currently, home care
workers are exempt from the Fair Labor Standards Act (FLSA), legislation passed in 1938 to "eliminate conditions detrimental to the maintenance of the minimum standard of living necessary for the health,
efficiency and general well-being of workers" (Biklen 2003). The FLSA
ensures that workers are given fair wages and compensation for overtime
work. Although the original act had little to say about domestic workers,
the legislation was amended in 1974 to extend coverage to domestic employees including home nurses, full-time nannies, chauffeurs, gardeners,
housekeepers, and cleaners. Home care workers as well as casual babysitters were excluded from this significant revision of the FLSA under what
is known as the "companionship exemption." Aides working in the home
were thought to provide "fellowship, care, and protection" of elderly or
disabled, work that Congress believed did not warrant protection under
federal law. Likening home care aides to casual babysitters, the law reinforced the legal boundary between paid labor and the intimate duties
of families (Biklen 2003), with the latter seen as outside the purview of
the state. In essence, aides were seen as doing the work of family, which,
as Congress viewed it, should "remain untouched by federal wage and
hour legislation" (Biklen 2003). Curiously, personal and home care aides
employed by third-party agencies (i.e., not the client) were also included in
the exemption, leaving unprotected nearly 1.4 million low-skilled workers
in home care (P. Smith 2009).

In June 2007, the U.S. Supreme Court heard the case *Long Island Care at
Home v. Evelyn Coke*. Evelyn Coke was a seventy-four-year-old Jamaican
immigrant from Queens who worked nearly twenty years as a home care
aide, often clocking twenty-four-hour shifts without overtime pay. She
sued her employer, arguing that they violated FLSA by failing to pay her
minimum wage and overtime for her work (P. Smith 2009). Specifically,
her case challenged the Department of Labor's inclusion of aides working
for third-party agencies in the companionship exemption. The Supreme

Court ruled unanimously that because Congress was unclear about the scope of the exemption, the DOL's interpretation of the law was "reasonable and entitled to judicial deference" (P. Smith 2009). In essence, the ruling instructed courts to defer to the Department of Labor because the original intention of Congress was unclear (Boris and Klein 2007).

Although the *Coke* ruling was certainly a setback for home care aides and their advocates, it may have ushered in a political, albeit piecemeal, solution to the problem of the companionship exemption (Boris and Klein 2007). As it stands, there are two viable ways in which the exemption could be modified. According to legal scholar Peggie Smith (2009, 5), Congress could propose legislation to amend the FSLA, or the Department of Labor—under the pressure and guidance of the executive branch—could revise the companionship exemption themselves. The first approach, reform via the legislature, has been proposed via the Fair Home Health Care Act (2007). The bill limits the companionship exemption to "casual" home care workers, those who perform care in an "irregular or intermittent" way, who don't work for an agency, and who log fewer than twenty hours per week. By extension, the law would exclude from exemption aides employed by agencies. Aides who live in with their clients would continue to be exempt, and aides who provide around-the-clock care would remain uncompensated for time sleeping. The Fair Home Health Care Act was referred to the House Committee on Education and Labor, and in October 2007 the Subcommittee on Workforce Protections held hearings to receive testimony from key stakeholders. While this particular bill may never make it out of committee, it is possible that the companionship exemption will at some point be challenged via the U.S. legislature.

The second option for resolving the companionship exemption relies on the willingness of the Department of Labor to revise the regulations. Positive steps were taken in this direction by President Clinton in 2001, only to be erased by the Bush administration soon after. Under the Clinton administration, the DOL explored three possible revisions to the companionship exemption, each of which attempted to specify exactly how much "fellowship" an aide would have to perform to be considered exempt under FLSA. The proposals ranged from the vague (companionship exemption applies if fellowship is a "significant part" of a worker's duties) to the specific (exemption applies only if the worker spends at least 80 percent of his or her time engaged in fellowship). The revisions proposed under

Clinton did not challenge the basic premise of the companionship exemption, but rather sought to narrow its reach. Advocates made the case that home care of "today" goes well beyond companionship and fellowship to include a range of medical and domestic services that should be protected under the FLSA.

Although the Clinton proposals were withdrawn under the Bush administration,[2] home care workers, with the help of key advocates, have renewed hope of working through the Department of Labor. In May 2009, the Direct Care Alliance (a nonprofit advocacy organization) and the House Labor and Working Families Caucus worked together to circulate in Congress a "Dear Colleague" letter addressed to Labor Secretary Hilda L. Solis requesting a change in the scope of the companionship exemption. It remains to be seen what will come of this symbolic action, since changes to the companionship exemption—either through the legislature or through the Department of Labor—depend on the political climate and leadership of the day.

From a sociological perspective, the problem with the companionship exemption is less that it includes workers whose scope of work extends beyond fellowship, and more that the labor of companionship, emotional in its dimensions, is not considered work worthy of federal protection. As Molly Biklen (2003) notes, the exemption reflects and codifies an ideological separation of home and work, reinforcing the idea that interpersonal bonds formed between caregivers and clients are extensions of family ties found in the private sphere. As such, companionship and fellowship are viewed as familial social obligations, not work. When aides perform this care, then, they are family substitutes, not laborers in the conventional sense (Biklen 2003).

Aides are unlikely to win protections armed only with epistemological critiques of the law, but there is some merit to engaging in a broader discussion about whether companionship constitutes work and, if not, why this is the case. If, as Arlie Hochschild (2003) has observed, we are seeing a trend toward "marketized private life," it becomes increasingly important to critically investigate the ways in which tasks formerly associated with the private sphere of the family are offered as paid labor in a service economy. Doing so will necessarily require thoughtful consideration of the rather arbitrary distinctions drawn between paid and unpaid work, especially when it comes to labor in the home.

For example, few would disagree that bathing and dressing a disabled client or changing soiled bed linens is work worthy of a wage. Other relational tasks associated with home care, by contrast, prove trickier to categorize. Is it work to listen to an elderly woman talk about her fears about dying? Is it work to comfort someone in pain? Is it work to take an elderly man to the park to feed the birds? While we lack clear answers to these questions, most people acknowledge there would be real consequences if aides weren't paid to perform these tasks: clients would suffer both physically and emotionally, families would be burdened financially and emotionally, and the costs of care would likely rise as people leaned disproportionately on institutional care. We seem to understand on some level that personal and home care work should be compensated, if for no other reason than to attract people to the job, but we are conflicted about how much value—in the form of monetary compensation—we should assign to the labor.

The data presented in this book suggest that aides also struggle to negotiate the complex social norms and feeling rules associated with paid labor in the home, viewing their work as familial rather than formal. Although some might view such a perspective as naive or uninformed, home care aides do see their relational work (emoting, listening, providing companionship) as integral to high-quality client care. They are very clear that companionship is the most important thing that they do, above cleaning house and providing personal care to clients. Workers and clients alike appear to benefit when aides prioritize the relational aspects of caregiving, rather than limiting their care to tasks that can be completed at "arm's length." Even though some aides struggle to define their relational commitments as work worthy of compensation, they are unequivocal that intimate ties with clients produce a sense of job satisfaction and dignity. Rather than taking this as further evidence of home care as familial in nature and therefore outside the realm of paid labor, it behooves us to push for a broader understanding of paid care work that unapologetically places companionship at center.

Reconceptualizing paid care work in a way that takes seriously the importance of relational ties and companionship requires adjustments to theory, research, and policy. Scholars of care work must continue to investigate instances of "marketized private life" (Hochschild 2003), such as home care, in an effort to move beyond dualistic thinking about home/

family and work/labor that mires the existing literature on care. As Lynet Uttal and Mary Tuominen (1999) so eloquently argue, certain kinds of paid care work, especially those where relational ties are of utmost importance to workers, are unique forms of labor, "distinct from traditional explanations of labor as work exchanged for wages" (759). Failure to recognize this leads to simplified readings of care work as either structurally exploitive or based on altruism and love. Such false distinctions are neither empirically informed nor theoretically useful, given what we know to be true about the complexity of careworkers' experiences.

On an applied level, we should be cautious when arguing, as some labor advocates have, that home care aides are "more than companions" and therefore entitled to the protections under the Fair Labor Standards Act. Instead, legal scholars, politicians, and advocates must push for a reconceptualization of *companionship as labor,* worthy of fair compensation and protection under labor law. Until the basic premise of the exemption clause of FLSA is challenged, workers will have to continually defend their work as "more than companionship," which not only violates their experiences as workers but reinforces the idea that care work—largely the work of women—is not in fact work.

Reconceptualizing care work and companionship as paid labor is but one step toward reorienting public priorities with respect to long-term care. Efforts to improve the working lives of home care aides will only go so far unless coupled with more comprehensive reforms to the U.S. health care system. As it stands, community-based long-term care is inadequate for both low-skilled providers and the clients who receive care.[3] On the provider side, greater commitment at the federal and state level to living wages, sufficient benefits, and better training would help ensure that home care workers approach their work with dignity and confidence. On the client or patient side, we must redouble our efforts to create options for community-based care so that working families—many of whom earn too much to qualify for Medicaid-waiver money but earn too little to pay out of pocket for an aide—can keep their loved ones at home without sacrificing quality of care. Just as we leave many Americans to fend for themselves with respect to purchasing and paying for health care, we have been equally slow to support the elderly and disabled who want to remain in their own homes. In addition to covering the uninsured and keeping down skyrocketing medical costs, priority must also be given to restructuring long-term care in a way that bolsters the direct care workforce and creates a comprehensive system of community-based care. True health care reform can be achieved only when we address the needs of the elderly, the disabled, and their paid caregivers.

Appendix

Methods

This book is the product of an inductive, grounded-theory approach to understanding the work experiences of home care aides (Strauss 1987; Strauss and Corbin 1990).[1] I began the study with the goal of observing and documenting the realities of paid caregiving, with the specific aim of understanding how workers perceive their social locations, specifically their positions as low-waged workers. As Lofland and Lofland (1995) suggest, field methods that include observation and in-depth interviewing lend themselves to "involvement and enmeshment" rather than "objectivity and distance" (17). As such, I set out to observe and interview home care workers as they provided care to clients, as well as during trainings, union meetings, and social gatherings. While the bulk of the data come from one-on-one interviews with aides, observing aides on the job allowed me to contextualize and corroborate individual accounts. More important, it is through direct observation of aides that I came to appreciate just how demanding the work is, both physically and emotionally.

This study draws on the experiences of home care aides in both California and Ohio. While it was personal circumstance (I moved from California to work in Ohio) that allowed for a multistate study, the comparison proved more than fortuitous. Examining the experiences of aides across two different states allows for an important check on both the validity and reliability of worker accounts. My findings suggest that worker experiences are remarkably similar across the two contexts, even though California appears—on the surface—to be a better place for home care aides to live and work when considering wages, benefits, and level of unionization. When aides describe their work, especially in its affective dimensions, there is little difference between aides in Ohio and California. The only notable difference between the two states is the racial and ethnic composition of the workforce. Home care aides in both states are predominantly white, but racial and ethnic minorities make up a greater percentage of the workforce in California. As a result, greater racial and ethnic diversity is reflected in the California sample.

This book focuses on home care workers employed by three organizations in California and Ohio. The California sample is drawn from a state-run home care agency, In-Home Supportive Services (IHSS), and a for-profit home health care company, It's For You Home Care in Central City. The Ohio sample is drawn from a private agency, Maximum Care, located in Middletown. Including both for-profit agencies and a state program allows for an examination of the way in which the public and private sector manage home care and the extent to which the work experiences of aides vary by context. Elderly and disabled clients served by the IHSS program are considered low income, and almost all qualify for some form of subsidized health coverage, generally through Medicaid.[2] In contrast, It's For You and Maximum Care attract a wider range of clients, some of whom rely on public assistance for care, and others who pay out of pocket. In both the for-profit and state-run agencies, aides have minimal training, although a subset of the sample are licensed certified nursing assistants (CNAs) or state tested nursing assistants (STNAs). Neither state requires certification or formal training as a condition of employment in home care.

Two methods were used to collect data in this qualitative study: in-depth interviews and field observations. In total, thirty-three home care workers were interviewed (twenty-three in California, ten in Ohio). In California, thirteen interviews were conducted with home care workers employed by

IHSS, and ten with aides working for It's For You. In Ohio, ten interviews were conducted with aides working for Maximum Care. In addition to the thirty-three home care aides, I also interviewed eight public health nurses and three social workers, all employed by IHSS and who work directly with home care aides to coordinate client services. Finally, I interviewed six managers of personal home care services to get a sense of how agencies view home care aides and their work.

The participants in the study live in Central City, California, or Middletown, Ohio, and range from twenty-eight to seventy-one years of age. The mean age of aides is forty-eight years, and 80 percent (twenty-six aides) report high school as their highest level of education. The racial composition of the twenty-three aides in California is as follows: seven white, six African American, five Latino (two of whom are citizens), two Asian Americans, two Asians who are not yet citizens, and one person who identified as mixed race (Asian and white). The Ohio sample is entirely white and female, but otherwise mirrors the California sample in terms of average age of worker and level of education. Of home care aides interviewed, twenty-eight are female and five are male. Of social workers, public health nurses, and agency administrators interviewed, only one is male (n = 17) and all are white.

Interview participants in both Ohio and California were recruited via convenience sampling. After receiving human subjects approval, I began interviewing IHSS public health nurses and social workers in March of 2002, when a social worker friend introduced me to several of her co-workers at IHSS. At the same time, I began attending regular training workshops and orientation meetings for IHSS home care workers. I recruited IHSS workers during trainings and meetings, after making a general announcement about my study and sending around a "sign-up sheet." I attended twenty IHSS trainings and five other IHSS caregiver events over a six-month period. These events yielded the thirteen interviews conducted with IHSS workers between 2002 and 2003. I simultaneously recruited ten It's For You workers over the phone from a list of aides obtained from the agency. Maximum Care workers were recruited via flyers placed in pay envelopes (aides contacted me directly in this case).

All home care workers in the sample were offered a twenty-dollar stipend to participate in the study. Although the convenience sample yielded a wide variety of caregivers, with a range of motivations and levels of commitment, the fact that I sampled caregivers from voluntary trainings and orientation meetings, and relied on self-selection of subjects, means that workers who take seriously their care responsibilities are likely to be overrepresented. That said, the token payment of twenty dollars helped ensure that a wide range of workers responded to my requests for participation, since the monetary compensation likely enticed aides who might not otherwise have participated and whose motivations for caregiving were manifold.

Semistructured interviews with home care aides, public health nurses, social workers, and administrators lasted anywhere from one to three hours, with the average lasting an hour and a half. The interviews were tape recorded and transcribed, although two respondents—one public health nurse and one home care worker—asked me not to tape the interview. Interviews with public health nurses and social workers took place immediately after I accompanied them on home visits, usually during lunch or after we returned to the IHSS office. Some of the interviews with aides occurred at their place of work (i.e., the client's home), but most preferred to meet in a public place like McDonald's or the public library. In a few interviews with IHSS workers, an elderly or disabled client was present during the interview, but I never formally questioned these clients, in compliance with the wishes of the agency administrators. Fifteen family providers (relatives paid a wage by IHSS to care for their own family) were also interviewed, but their accounts and experiences are not included in the present analysis.[3]

During interviews with home care workers, I inquired how they became caregivers; whether they became caregivers by choice, by obligation, or by economic necessity; and whether they felt a sense of autonomy or empowerment in their work. I also asked them to describe both the constraints and rewards of paid caregiving. I posed a similar set of questions to public health nurses and social workers, in addition to inviting them to speak at length about working alongside home care aides. When interviewing agency administrators, I focused on staffing constraints and their experiences managing aides.

In conjunction with interviews, I spent the first six months of the study (March–September 2002) observing care "on-site," approximately ten hours a week. I accompanied public health nurses and social workers to the homes of elderly and disabled clients. Tagging along on "ride arounds" allowed me to directly observe home care and assess how caregiving responsibilities are shared with nurses, social workers, and the client's family. Most of the ethnographic observations discussed in the book come from this early and intensive period of field observations, although I did continue to observe aides on-site even as my attention turned to one-on-one interviews.[4]

Initially it was difficult to develop a rapport with the home care aides during trainings and interviews as some suspected me of being a social worker and therefore a county employee "spying" on them. This misunderstanding largely stemmed from confusion on the part of the respondents about the distinction between a social worker and a sociologist. After several interviews, I learned to introduce myself as an independent researcher first, and a sociologist second. This seemed to dispel the misunderstanding that I somehow worked for the county. After several months of being in the field, I was no longer an "outsider" and found that caregivers would greet me as a friend or acquaintance when we would encounter one another at trainings or events. More often than not, caregivers generously opened up their homes (or places of work) to me, even if they were in the middle of tending to a parent, child, or client. Several home care workers fed me, while others spent time showing me family albums or giving me a tour of their home or workplace.

My social location as a middle-class, educated, white researcher was certainly a factor in my interactions with home care workers. I found that while the topic of race and racism occasionally made for uncomfortable conversation for respondents, few caregivers shied away from the topic altogether. In general, caregivers were very open about their experiences and feelings pertaining to care. Probably because their work can be very isolating, lonely, and sometimes depressing, the caregivers I met were eager to have someone to listen to their stories. In Ohio, a few of the respondents actively sought out inclusion in the study after hearing about me from a fellow aide. A handful of aides, in both California and Ohio, expressed gratitude after an interview, seeming incredulous that someone had taken an interest in their work. This expression of gratitude surprised me as I generally felt a nuisance for asking a favor from people who had little time to themselves or their families. I think, however, that I had, in my initial assumptions, arrogantly underestimated the importance of a sense of dignity in relation to one's work, irrespective of where one falls on the occupational ladder. As Randy Hodson (2001) so astutely puts it, "Life demands dignity, and meaningful work is essential for dignity."

NOTES

Introduction

1. The pseudonyms of Central City, Middletown, It's For You, and Maximum Care are used to protect the confidentiality of research subjects. The names and identifiers of organizations and informants are kept confidential in accordance with federal and university human subjects procedures. This project received initial human subjects approval in January 2002, and approval was renewed annually through 2009.

2. Home care aides are exempt from the Fair Labor Standards Act (FLSA), legislation that ensures fair wages and overtime protection for workers. Under the "companionship exemption" of the FLSA (1974), home care aides are not granted protections afforded other domestic workers because they provide "fellowship, care and protection" to the elderly or disabled, work that Congress does not believe warrants federal protection. To justify the exemption, Congress argued that home care aides, like babysitters, do the "intimate work of families," which is beyond the purview (and therefore the legal protections) of the state. Advocacy groups such as the Direct Care Alliance have in the last ten years launched campaigns to eliminate the companionship exemption, arguing that home care aides engage in demanding physical labor and are therefore "more than companions" to their clients. Aides do not, as one advocate wrote in a newsletter, "sit and watch *The Price Is Right* with consumers" (Hanson 2010).

3. Both the Paraprofessional Healthcare Institute (New York) and the Center for Personal Assistance Services (University of California, San Francisco) refer to home care aides as personal and home care workers.

4. Medicare reimburses for short-term home health care but does not pay for longer-term, custodial care of elderly or disabled adults.

1. The Costs of Caring

1. The Bureau of Labor Statistics reports that nurse aides have the highest incidence rate of workplace injuries and illnesses in the country (Paraprofessional Healthcare Institute 2008a), which belies aides' assertions that they "don't get sick." Perhaps a more accurate characterization is that aides simply don't seek treatment when ill because they lack the insurance to do so.

2. Medicaid waiver programs give states discretion to develop and fund home- and community-based programs for the elderly and disabled, as an alternative to institutionalization.

2. Doing the Dirty Work

1. In the last twenty years, service unions have led a series of successful campaigns to organize allied health workers, including home care aides, recognizing the critical importance of this labor force for maintaining labor's longevity in the postindustrial era (Boris and Klein 2006; Ducey 2009). Training and the "upgrading of jobs" are now signature components of the organizing strategies of unions that represent health care workers, as are some of the "benefits" unions offer their rank and file once organized (Ducey 2009). While laudable, training programs, as Ariel Ducey notes, fail to address the more systemic problems in the organization of health care that indirectly, but detrimentally, affect workers, such as inattention to care for the chronically ill (and, I would add, inattention to long-term care services) and a generally "fractured" health care system (Ducey 2009, 6).

2. The potential for exploitation of workers in home care is not unlike the exploitation identified by Judith Rollins in her classic work, *Between Women* (1985). Rollins's study of black domestics working for white middle-class women suggests that exploitation is often embedded in work where intimate social relationships are central (such as domestic labor). She writes, "What might appear to be the basis of a more humane, less alienating work arrangement allows for a level of psychosocial exploitation unknown in other occupations" (156). Home care work certainly has the potential to be exploitative, and many aides describe arrangements that are physically, emotionally, or economically harmful to them. Home care differs from domestic work in a couple important ways, however. Clients in home care are often themselves disenfranchised by age or illness, which means they occupy very different social locations from the middle- and upper-class women and men who hire domestics. Second, there is a presumption of intimacy in home care (on the part of client and caregiver) that comes from crossing boundaries of personal space (aides, for example, can be called on to change clients' diapers, wash their bodies, or brush their teeth). Home care is thus qualitatively different from other kinds of domestic work in terms of the relationships formed with "employers" (clients) and the emotional labor required.

3. The Rewards of Caring

1. Michele Lamont, in *The Dignity of Working Men* (2000), also uses the term "caring self," in reference to the boundary work that black workers engage in to distance themselves from "domineering" white workers. Although my use of "caring self" here is a more general exploration of identity work across racial groups in a given occupation (home care), I find Lamont's theorization of the caring self relevant to the present discussion of identity work performed by aides of color. Like the black men in Lamont's study, the black, Latino, and Filipino home care workers from Middletown and Central City profess a superior caring self relative to white women in the same field.

2. Jaxon VanDerbeken, "Woman and Caregiver Die in Apparent Suicide Pact," *San Francisco Chronicle,* January 10, 2006.

3. In her study of family child care workers, Tuominen (1998) also finds that African American women consciously affirm their racial and ethnic identities by providing much needed care to children and families within their own communities.

4. Organizing Home Care

1. In 1999, seventy-four thousand IHSS home care workers in Los Angeles County elected to join SEIU's Local 434B, arguably the most impressive victory for organized labor since 1941 (Delp and Quan 2002).

2. In late 2008, *Los Angeles Times* reporter Paul Pringle broke the story of Tyrone Freeman, president of SEIU Local 6434, accused of misappropriating approximately $1 million in union funds. Freeman allegedly channeled the money to his wife's day care and home-based video businesses, while also spending union funds on a golf tournament and expensive outings at restaurants and cigar lounges. Former SEIU President Andy Stern imposed a lifetime ban on Freeman and ordered him to repay the misappropriated money (Paul Pringle, "Service Union Bans Former California Local President for Life," *Los Angeles Times,* December 27, 2008). In early 2009, the escalating feud between United Healthcare Workers-West in Oakland and SEIU leadership culminated when SEIU ousted UHW's local president, Sal Rosselli, and placed the chapter into trusteeship. Rosselli subsequently formed a new organization, National Union of Healthcare Workers, which seeks to draw membership from SEIU's rank and file. The initial disagreement between Rosselli and SEIU stems from Stern's proposal to transfer sixty-five thousand of UHW's members into a different chapter as part of a larger consolidation effort. Rosselli and his supporters argued that such mergers would result in a less democratic union for workers (Paul Pringle, "Breakaway Union Could Prompt War of Attrition with SEIU," *Los Angeles Times,* February 2, 2009). National Union of Healthcare Workers continues its campaign to recruit current and prospective rank and file from SEIU, holding decertification elections and organizing campaigns throughout California.

3. The executive order signed by Strickland suggests possible cooperation of the state with respect to the collective bargaining of home care aides in Ohio, although such "friendships" are fragile and depend largely on the political persuasion of those in power. Unless codified by legislation, executive orders have a tendency to blow with the political wind.

4. Over the last thirty years, aides working for private and nonprofit agencies in New York have slowly organized with the help of SEIU 1199 and AFSCME. As part of the "Campaign for Justice" that began in the 1980s, union leaders engaged in direct political action and forged alliances with key stakeholders—such as political leaders and home care agency owners—to ultimately win higher wages and better benefits for aides (Mareschal 2006). Political elite in New York, for example, benefited from generous campaign contributions from SEIU in exchange for their support of workers. Those who proposed cuts in public funding for home care or who opposed unionization found themselves ostracized publicly by a very active and politically savvy local. Perhaps more importantly, 1199 and AFSCME worked with the Home Care Council of New York, which represented the interests of sixty nonprofit agencies, to successfully lobby state authorities to increase reimbursement to agencies. This alliance with agency subcontractors continued into the new millennium when, during a 2004 strike in New York City, agencies allowed unionization of their workers with the assurance that SEIU would put resources and energy behind a campaign to increase state funding for home care (Mareschal 2006). It remains to be seen whether SEIU (or any other union, for that matter) will be able to form similar meaningful alliances with politicians and/or home care agencies in Ohio. The fact that Governor Strickland signed an executive order in 2007 granting collective bargaining rights to independent home health workers suggests that there are potential allies at the state level.

5. I interviewed a small number of paid family caregivers (fourteen), employed by IHSS, who were active in the union in Central City. Family providers are paid by the state to care for their own relatives and constitute about 40 percent of the total number of aides working for IHSS in California (Holgate and Shea 2006). Because the work of family providers is qualitatively different from that of aides who are unrelated to clients, their accounts are not included in this chapter's discussion of unionization, nor are they discussed in the book.

6. Disputes within and between different factions of the labor movement continue to plague organized labor. In 2005, Andrew Stern, president of SEIU, precipitated a split of several service unions (including SEIU) from AFL-CIO to form a new federation, Change to Win. Since that time, intralabor tension has increased as unions vie for membership, often competing aggressively with one another to win jurisdiction over a given industry or region (Steven Greenhouse, "Infighting Distracts Unions at Crucial Time," *New York Times,* July 8, 2009). Recent scandals involving SEIU in California have only intensified fissures within the labor movement.

Conclusion

1. In 2010, New York passed legislation guaranteeing basic rights and protections for nannies, housekeepers, and caregivers in the state. The Domestic Workers Bill of Rights, the first of its kind in U.S. history, mandates overtime wages and paid leave for workers generally excluded from federal labor laws. California and Colorado are considering similar legislation (Russ Buettner, "For Nannies, Hope for Workplace Protection," *New York Times,* June 2, 2010).

2. Many argue that extending FLSA protection to home care workers would raise the costs of care for agencies, thereby reducing services for elderly and disabled clients. Similar claims were used by the Bush administration to justify their opposition to FLSA protection for aides (Boris and Klein 2007).

3. The health care reform legislation signed into law in March 2010 (Patient Protection and Affordable Care Act) contains a long-term care provision known as the Community Living Assistance Services and Support (CLASS) Act. While the details of this provision have not been fully specified, it appears that working individuals enrolled in the insurance program will be eligible for long-term care benefits of up to seventy-five dollars per day (average monthly premiums are projected to be $123). This legislation, championed initially by the late Senator Edward Kennedy, will potentially help offset the costs of long-term care for many working people. Importantly, CLASS does not exclude people with preexisting health conditions from enrollment. The legislation takes effect January 1, 2011, but enrollment will not begin until 2013 (Paula Span, "Details on the Class Act," *New York Times,* April 29, 2010).

Appendix

1. I draw on mainstream sociological approaches to the collection and analysis of qualitative data. Specifically, I write in the tradition of interpretive sociology, which aims to "study things in their natural settings, attempting to make sense of, or interpret, phenomena in terms of the meanings people bring to them" (Denzin and Lincoln 1998). Interpretative sociology claims roots in the Chicago School and the symbolic interactionist work of scholars such as George Herbert Mead, Everett Hughes, and Howard Becker. Interpretivists often (though not always) employ grounded theory when collecting and analyzing data, an inductive approach that allows the researcher to generate social theory *from* the empirical world, rather than testing hypotheses *in* the empirical world (Denzin and Lincoln 1998).

2. Medicare (Title XIII) and Medicaid (Title XIX) are together known as the Social Security Amendments of 1965. Medicaid provides broad health coverage to low-income individuals and, in both California and Ohio, offers in-home services to elderly or disabled adults through

Medicaid-waiver programs. Medicare, in contrast, does not provide home-based, long-term care services to the elderly or disabled.

3. For analysis of IHSS family providers, see Clare Stacey and Lindsey Ayers, "Stigmatized Labors: The Experiences of Paid Family Caregivers" (unpublished manuscript, Kent, OH, 2011).

4. Ethnographic observations are of California workers only; Ohio data are based on interviews.

References

Aronson, Jane. 1992. "Women's Sense of Responsibility for the Care of Old People: But Who Else Is Going to Do It?" *Gender and Society* 6 (1): 8–29.

Ashforth, Blake E., and Ronald H. Humphrey. 1993. "Emotional Labor in Service Roles: The Influence of Identity." *Academy of Management Review* 18 (1): 108–15.

Ashforth, Blake E., and Glen E. Kreiner. 1999. "How Can You Do It? Dirty Work and the Challenge of Constructing a Positive Identity." *Academy of Management Review* 24 (3): 413–34.

Ashforth, Blake E., Glen E. Kreiner, Mark A. Clark, and Mel Fugate. 2007. "Normalizing Dirty Work: Managerial Tactics for Countering Occupational Taint." *Academy of Management Journal* 50 (1): 149–74.

Benjamin, A. E. 1993. "An Historical Perspective on Home Care Policy." *Milbank Quarterly* 71 (1): 129–66.

Benjamin, A. E., Ruth Matthias, and Todd M. Franke. 2000. "Comparing Consumer-Directed and Agency Models for Providing Supportive Services at Home." *Health Services Research* 35 (1): 351–66.

Berdes, Celia, and John M. Eckert. 2007. "The Language of Caring: Nurse's Aides' Use of Family Metaphors Conveys Affective Care." *Gerontologist* 47 (3): 340–49.

Berg, Gretchen, and Susan Farrar. 2000. *IHSS Providers: Characteristics of Caregivers in the In-Home Supportive Services Program.* Sacramento: California Department of Social Services.

Biklen, Molly. 2003. "Healthcare in the Home: Reexamining the Companionship Services Exemption to the Fair Labor Standards Act." *Columbia Human Rights Law Review* 113.

Bird, Chloe E., and Patricia P. Rieker. 2008. *Gender and Health: The Effects of Constrained Choices and Social Policies.* Cambridge: Cambridge University Press.

Boris, Eileen, and Jennifer Klein. 2006. "Organizing Home Care: Low-Waged Workers in the Welfare State." *Politics and Society* 34 (1): 81–107.

——. 2007. "Laws of Care: The Supreme Court and Aides to Elderly People." *Dissent* (Fall): 128–30.

Brannon, Diane, Jacqueline S. Zinn, Vincent Mor, and Jullet Davis. 2002. "An Exploration of Job, Organizational, and Environmental Factors Associated with High and Low Nursing Assistant Turnover." *Gerontologist* 42 (2): 159–68.

Bureau of Labor Statistics. 2005. *Occupational Outlook Handbook 2005–2006.* Washington, DC: U.S. Department of Labor.

——. 2009. *Occupational Employment Statistics Survey (May): Personal and Home Care Aides.* Washington, DC: U.S. Department of Labor.

——. 2010. Occupational Outlook Handbook 2009–2010. Washington, DC: U.S. Department of Labor.

Cahill, Spencer. 1999. "Emotional Capital and Professional Socialization: The Case of Mortuary Science Students (and Me)." *Social Psychology Quarterly* 62 (2): 101–16.

Calasanti, Toni M., and Kathleen F. Slevin. 2001. *Gender, Social Inequalities, and Aging.* Walnut Creek, CA: AltaMira Press.

California Association of Public Authorities for IHSS. 2010. "Who We Are." http://www.capaihss.org.

California Welfare Directors Association. 2002. *In-Home Supportive Services: Past, Present and Future.* Sacramento: Adult Services Committee, CWDA.

Cancian, Francesca M., and Stacey J. Oliker. 2001. *Caring and Gender.* Walnut Creek, CA: AltaMira Press.

Chambliss, Daniel F. 1996. *Beyond Caring: Hospitals, Nurses and the Social Organization of Ethics.* Chicago: University of Chicago Press.

Chechin, Eileen R. 1993. "Home Care Is Where the Heart Is: The Role of Interpersonal Relationships in Paraprofessional Home Care." *Home Health Care Services Quarterly* 13 (1): 161–77.

Chodorow, Nancy. 1978. *The Reproduction of Mothering.* Berkeley: University of California Press.

Clawson, Dan. 2003. *The Next Upsurge: Labor and New Social Movements.* Ithaca, NY: Cornell University Press.

Conradson, David. 2003. "Geographies of Care: Spaces, Practices, Experiences." *Social and Cultural Geography* 4 (4): 451–54.

Crown, William H., Dennis A. Ahlburg, and Margaret MacAdam. 1995. "The Demographic and Employment Characteristics of Home Care Aides: A Comparison with Nursing Home Aides, Hospital Aides, and Other Workers." *Gerontologist* 35 (2): 162–71.

Davies, Celia. 1995. "Competence Versus Care? Gender and Caring Work Revisited." *Acta Sociologica* 38: 17–31.

Delp, Linda, and Katie Quan. 2002. "Homecare Worker Organizing in California: An Analysis of a Successful Strategy." *Labor Studies Journal* 27 (1): 1–23.

Denzin, Norman K., and Yvonna S. Lincoln. 1998. *The Landscape of Qualitative Research*. Thousand Oaks, CA: Sage.

Diamond, Timothy. 1992. *Making Gray Gold: Narratives of Nursing Home Care*. Chicago: University of Chicago Press.

Doka, Kenneth J. 1989. *Disenfranchised Grief*. Lexington, MA: Lexington Books.

Drew, Shirley K., Melanie B. Mills, and Bob M. Gassaway. 2007. *Dirty Work: The Social Construction of Taint*. Waco, TX: Baylor University Press.

Ducey, Ariel. 2009. *Never Good Enough: Health Care Workers and the False Promise of Job Training*. Ithaca, NY: Cornell University Press.

Duffy, Mignon. 2005. "Reproducing Labor Inequalities: Challenges for Feminists Conceptualizing Care at the Intersections of Gender, Race and Class." *Gender and Society* 19 (1): 66–82.

———. 2007. "Doing the Dirty Work: Gender, Race and Reproductive Labor in Historical Perspective." *Gender and Society* 21 (3): 313–37.

Edin, Kathryn, and Laura Lein. 1997. *Making Ends Meet: How Single Mothers Survive Welfare and Low-Wage Work*. New York: Russell Sage Foundation.

Ehrenreich, Barbara, and Arlie Russell Hochschild. 2002. *Global Woman: Nannies, Maids, and Sex Workers in the New Economy*. New York: Metropolitan Books.

Ejaz, Farida, Linda Noelker, Heather Menne, and Joshua Bagaka. 2008. "The Impact of Stress and Support on Direct Care Workers' Job Satisfaction." *Gerontologist* 48 (1): 60–70.

England, Paula, Michelle Budig, and Nancy Folbre. 2002. "Wages of Virtue: The Relative Pay of Care Work." *Social Problems* 49 (4): 455–73.

Erickson, Rebecca J. 1995. "The Importance of Authenticity for Self and Society." *Symbolic Interaction* 18 (2): 121–44.

Erickson, Rebecca J., and Wendy J. C. Grove. 2007. "Why Emotion Matters: Age Agitation and Burnout among Registered Nurses." *Online Journal of Issues in Nursing* 13 (1). http://www.nursingworld.org/MainMenuCategories/ANAMarketplace/ANAPeriodicals/OJIN/TableofContents/vol132008/No1Jan08/ArticlePrevious Topic/WhyEmotionsMatterAgeAgitationandBurnoutAmongRegisteredNurses. aspx.

———. 2008. "Emotional Labor and Health Care." *Sociology Compass* 2 (2): 704–33.

Erickson, Rebecca J., and Amy S. Wharton. 1997. "Inauthenticity and Depression: Assessing the Consequences of Interactive Service Work." *Work and Occupations* 24 (2): 188–213.

Feagin, Joe R., and Melvin P. Sikes. 1994. *Living with Racism: The Black Middle Class Experience*. Boston: Beacon Press.

Folbre, Nancy. 2001. *The Invisible Heart: Economics and Family Values*. New York: New Press.

Foner, Nancy. 1994. *The Caregiving Dilemma: Work in an American Nursing Home*. Berkeley: University of California Press.

Goffman, Erving. 1963. *Stigma: Notes on the Management of Spoiled Identity*. Englewood Cliffs, NJ: Prentice-Hall.

Gordon, Suzanne, Patricia Benner, and Nel Noddings. 1996. *Caregiving: Readings in Knowledge, Practice, Ethics and Politics.* Philadelphia: University of Pennsylvania Press.

Gutek, Barbara A., Bennett Cherry, Anita D. Bhappu, Sherry Schneider, and Loren Woolf. 2000. "Features of Service Relationships and Encounters." *Work and Occupations* 27 (3): 319–51.

Hanson, Helen. 2010. "More Than a Companion: My Visit to the Department of Labor." *Direct Care News.* New York: Direct Care Alliance.

Harrington Meyer, Madonna. 2000. *Care Work: Gender, Labor and the Welfare State.* New York: Routledge.

Harris-Kojetin, Lauren, Debra Lipson, Jean Fielding, Kristen Kiefer, and Robyn I. Stone. 2004. *Recent Findings on Frontline Long-Term Care Workers: A Research Synthesis 1999–2003.* Washington, DC: Institute for the Future of Aging Services.

Himmelweit, Susan. 1999. "Caring Labor." *Annals of the American Academy* 561 (1): 27–38.

Hochschild, Arlie. 1979. "Emotion Work, Feeling Rules, and Social Structure." *American Journal of Sociology* 85 (3): 551–75.

———. 1983. *The Managed Heart: Commercialization of Human Feeling.* Berkeley: University of California Press.

———. 2003. *The Managed Heart: Twentieth Anniversary Edition.* Berkeley: University of California Press.

Hodson, Randy. 2001. *Dignity at Work.* Cambridge: Cambridge University Press.

Holgate, Brandynn, and Jennifer Shea. 2006. "SEIU Confronts the Home Care Crisis in California. New Politics 11 (1). http://www.wpunj.edu/newpol/issue41/Shea Holgate41.htm.

Hollander Feldman, Penny. 1994. "Dead End Work or Motivating Job? Prospects for Frontline Paraprofessional Workers in LTC." *Generations* 18 (3): 5–10.

Holstein, James A., and Jaber F. Gubrium. 2000. *The Self We Live By: Narrative Identity in a Postmodern World.* Oxford: Oxford University Press.

Hondagneu-Sotelo, Pierrette. 2001. *Domestica: Immigrant Workers Cleaning and Caring in the Shadows of Affluence.* Berkeley: University of California Press.

Howes, Candace. 2004. *Upgrading California's Home Care Workforce: The Impact of Political Action and Unionization.* Berkeley: Institute for Research on Labor and Employment, University of California.

———. 2005. "Living Wages and Retention of Homecare Workers in San Francisco." *Industrial Relations* 44 (1): 139–63.

———. 2006. *Building a High Quality Home Care Workforce: Wages, Benefits and Flexibility Matter.* Washington, DC: Robert Wood Johnson Foundation.

———. 2008. "Love, Money, or Flexibility: What Motivates People to Work in Consumer-Directed Home Care?" *Gerontologist* 48 (Suppl. 1): 46–59.

Hughes, Everett C. 1971. *The Sociological Eye: Selected Papers.* Chicago: Aldine Atherton.

Ibarra, Maria de la Luz. 2000. "Mexican Immigrant Women and the New Domestic Labor." *Human Organization* 59 (4): 452–65.

———. 2002. "Emotional Proletarians in a Global Economy: Mexican Immigrant Women and Elder Care Work." *Urban Anthropology and Studies of Cultural Systems and World Economic Development* 31 (3–4): 317–51.

Illouz, Eva. 1997. "Who Will Care for the Caretaker's Daughter? Towards a Sociology of Happiness in the Era of Reflexive Modernity." *Theory, Culture and Society* 14 (4): 31–66.

——. 2007. *Cold Intimacies: The Making of Emotional Capitalism*. Cambridge: Polity Press.

Institute of Medicine of the National Academies. 2008. *Retooling for an Aging America: Building the Healthcare Workforce*. Washington, DC: Institute of Medicine.

Jacobs, Jerry, and Kathleen Gerson. 2004. *The Time Divide: Work, Family, and Gender Inequality*. Cambridge, MA: Harvard University Press.

Karner, Tracy. 1998. "Professional Caring: Homecare Workers as Fictive Kin." *Journal of Aging Studies* 12 (1): 69–73.

Katz Rothman, Barbara. 1983. "Midwives in Transition: The Structure of a Clinical Revolution." *Social Problems* 30 (3): 262–71.

Kaye, Stephen, Susan Chapman, Robert Newcomer, and Charlene Harrington. 2006. "The Personal Assistance Workforce: Trends in Supply and Demand." *Health Affairs* 25 (4): 1113–20.

Kemper, Peter, Brigitt Heier, Teta Barry, Diane Brannon, Joe Angelelli, Joe Vasey, and Mindy Anderson-Knott. 2008. "What Do Direct Care Workers Say Would Improve Their Jobs? Differences across Settings." *Gerontologist* 48 (Suppl. 1): 17–25.

Lamont, Michele. 2000. *The Dignity of Working Men: Morality and the Boundaries of Race, Class, and Immigration*. Cambridge, MA: Harvard University Press.

Lan, Pei-Chia. 2002. "Subcontracting Filial Piety: Elder Care in Ethnic Chinese Immigrant Families in California." *Journal of Family Issues* 23 (7): 812–35.

Leidner, Robin. 1991. "Serving Hamburgers and Selling Insurance: Gender, Work, and Identity in Interactive Service Jobs." *Gender and Society* 5 (2): 154–77.

——. 1993. *Fast Food, Fast Talk: Service Work and the Routinization of Everyday Life*. Berkeley: University of California Press.

——. 1999. "Emotional Labor in Service Work." *The Annals of the American Academy* 561 (1): 81–95.

Lofland, Lyn, and John Lofland. 1995. *Analyzing Social Settings: A Guide to Qualitative Observation and Analysis*. Belmont, CA: Wadsworth.

Lopez, Steven H. 2004. *Reorganizing the Rust Belt: An Inside Study of the American Labor Movement*. Berkeley: University of California Press.

——. 2006. "Emotional Labor and Organized Emotional Care." *Work and Occupations* 33 (2): 133–60.

Lovell, Terry. 2000. "Thinking Feminism with and against Bourdieu." *Feminist Theory* 1 (1): 11–32.

Macdonald, Cameron L. 2010. *Shadow Mothers: Nannies, Au Pairs, and the Micropolitics of Mothering*. Berkeley: University of California.

Macdonald, Cameron L., and Carmen Sirianni. 1996. *Working in the Service Society*. Philadelphia: Temple University Press.

Mareschal, Patrice M. 2006. "Innovation and Adaptation: Contrasting Efforts to Organize Home Care Workers in Four States." *Labor Studies Journal* 31 (1): 25–49.

——. 2007. "How the West Was Won: An Inside View of the SEIU's Strategies and Tactics for Organizing Home Care Workers in Oregon." *International Journal of Organization Theory and Behavior* 10 (3): 386–412.

Mills, C. Wright. 1940. "Situated Actions and Vocabularies of Motive." *American Sociological Review* 5 (6): 904–13.

Mitchell, Daniel J. B. 2004. *Recent Developments in California Labor Relations.* Berkeley: Institute for Labor and Employment.

Montgomery, Rhonda J. V., Lyn Holley, Jerome Deichert, and Karl Kosloski. 2005. "A Profile of Home Care Workers from the 2000 Census: How It Changes What We Know." *Gerontologist* 45 (5): 593–600.

Moreton, Bethany. 2009. *To Serve God and Walmart: The Making of Christian Free Enterprise.* Cambridge, MA: Harvard University Press.

Munger, Frank, ed. 2002. *Laboring below the Line: The New Ethnography of Poverty, Low-Wage Work and Survival in the Global Economy.* New York: Russell Sage Foundation.

Muntaner, Carles. 2006. "Work Organization, Economic Inequality, and Depression among Nursing Assistants: A Multilevel Modeling Approach." *Psychological Reports* 98 (2): 585–601.

Muntaner, Carles, Yong Li, Xiaonan Xue, Theresa Thompson, HaeJoo Chung, and Patricia O'Campo. 2006. "County and Organizational Predictors of Depression Symptoms among Low-Income Nursing Assistants." *Social Science and Medicine* 63 (4): 1454–65.

Nakano Glenn, Evelyn. 1992. "From Servitude to Service Work: Historical Continuities in the Racial Division of Paid Reproductive Labor." *Signs* 18 (1): 1–43.

———. 2000. "Creating a Caring Society." *Contemporary Sociology* 29 (1): 84–94.

National Center on Elder Abuse. 1998. *National Elder Abuse Incidence Study: Final Report.* N.p.: American Public Human Services Association/Westat.

Newman, Katherine S. 1999a. *A Different Shade of Gray: Midlife and Beyond in the Inner City.* New York: Vintage.

———. 1999b. *No Shame in My Game: The Working Poor in the Inner City.* New York: Alfred A. Knopf and Russell Sage Foundation.

Neysmith, Sheila, and Jane Aronson. 1996. "Home Care Workers Discuss Their Work: The Skills Required to 'Use Your Common Sense.'" *Journal of Aging Studies* 10 (1): 1–4.

Nowotny, Helga. 1981. "Women in Public Life in Austria." In *Access to Power: Cross-National Studies of Women and Elites,* ed. C. F. Epstein and R. L. Coser, 147–56. London: George Allen and Unwin.

Ong, Paul, Jordan Rickles, Ruth Matthias, and A. E. Benjamin. 2002. *California Caregivers: Final Labor Market Analysis.* Los Angeles: UCLA School of Public Policy and Social Research.

Paraprofessional Healthcare Institute. 2008a. *The Invisible Care Gap: Ten Key Facts.* New York: PHI.

———. 2008b. *Occupational Projections for Direct Care Workers 2006–2016.* New York: PHI.

———. 2008c. *State Chart Book on Wages for Personal and Home Care Aides, 1999–2006.* New York: PHI.

Parks, Jennifer A. 2003. *No Place Like Home? Feminist Ethics and Home Health Care.* Bloomington: Indiana University Press.

Parrenas, Rhacel Salazar. 2001. *Servants of Globalization: Women, Migration and Domestic Work*. Stanford: Stanford University Press.

Paules, Greta Foff. 1991. *Dishing It Out: Power and Resistance among Waitresses in a New Jersey Restaurant*. Philadelphia: Temple University Press.

Potter, Sharyn J., Allison Churilla, and Kristin Smith. 2006. "An Examination of Full-Time Employment in the Direct-Care Workforce." *Journal of Applied Gerontology* 25 (5): 356–74.

Reay, Diane. 2004. "Gendering Bourdieu's Concepts of Capitals? Emotional Capital, Women and Social Class." *Sociological Review* 53 (1): 57–74.

Reinhard, Susan. 2001. *Consumer Directed Care and Nurse Practice Acts*. New Brunswick, NJ: Institute for Health, Healthcare Policy, and Aging Research.

Rollins, Judith. 1985. *Between Women: Domestics and Their Employers*. Philadelphia: Temple University.

Romero, Mary. 1992. *Maid in the U.S.A.* New York: Routledge.

Roth, Julius. 1963. *Timetables: Structuring the Passage of Time in Hospital Treatment and Other Careers*. Indianapolis: Bobbs-Merrill.

Scherzer, Teresa, and Nicole Wolfe. 2008. "Barriers to Workers' Compensation and Medical Care for Injured Personal Assistance Service Workers." *Home Health Care Services Quarterly* 27 (1): 37–58.

Seavey, Dorie. 2004. *The Cost of Frontline Turnover in Long-Term Care*. Washington, DC: Institute for Aging Services/American Association of Homes and Services for the Aging.

Sherman, Rachel. 2007. *Class Acts: Service and Inequality in Luxury Hotels*. Berkeley: University of California Press.

Smith, Kristin, and Reagan Baughman. 2007a. "Caring for America's Aging Population: A Profile of the Direct-Care Workforce." *Monthly Labor Review* 130 (9): 20–26.

———. 2007b. "Low Wage Prevalent in Direct Care and Childcare Workforces." Policy Brief no. 7, Casey Institute.

Smith, Peggie. 2009. *Protecting Home Care Workers under the Fair Labor Standards Act*. New York: Direct Care Alliance.

Smith, Vicki. 1998. "The Fractured World of the Temporary Worker: Power, Participation, and Fragmentation in the Contemporary Workplace." *Social Problems* 45:411–30.

———. 2001. *Crossing the Great Divide: Worker Risk and Opportunity in the New Economy*. Ithaca, NY: Cornell University Press, ILR.

Smith, Vicki, and Esther B. Neuwirth. 2008. *The Good Temp*. Ithaca, NY: Cornell University Press, ILR.

Snow, David, and Leon Anderson. 1987. "Identity Work among Homeless: The Verbal Construction and Avowal of Personal Identities." *American Journal of Sociology* 92 (6): 1336–72.

Solari, Cinzia. 2006. "Professionals and Saints: How Immigrant Careworkers Negotiate Gender Identities at Work." *Gender and Society* 20 (3): 301–31.

Spenner, Kenneth I., Luther B. Otto, and Vaughn R. A. Call. 1982. *Career Lines and Careers*. Lexington, MA: Lexington Books.

Stack, Carol B. 1974. *All Our Kin: Strategies for Survival in a Black Community*. New York: Harper and Row.

Steinberg, Ronnie J., and Deborah M. Figart. 1999. "Emotional Labor since *The Managed Heart." Annals of the American Academy* 561 (1): 8–26.

Stone, Deborah. 2000a. "Caring by the Book." In *Carework: Gender, Labor and the Welfare State,* ed. M. H. Meyers, 89–111. New York: Routledge.

———. 2000b. *Long-Term Care for the Elderly with Disabilities: Current Policy, Emerging Trends and Implications for the Twenty-First Century.* New York: Milbank Memorial Fund.

Stone, Pamela. 2007. *Opting Out? Why Women Really Quit Careers and Head Home.* Berkeley: University of California.

Stone, Robyn I. 2001. "Research on Frontline Workers in Long-Term Care." *Generations* 25 (1): 49–57.

———. 2004. "The Direct Care Worker: A Key Dimension of Home Care Policy." *Home Health Care Management and Practice* 16 (5): 339–49.

Stone, Robyn I., and Joshua M. Wiener. 2001. *Who Will Care For Us? Addressing the Long-Term Care Workforce Crisis.* Washington, DC: The Urban Institute, American Association of Homes and Services for Aging, and Robert Wood Johnson.

Strauss, Anselm. 1987. *Qualitative Analysis for Social Scientists.* New York: Cambridge University Press.

Strauss, Anselm, and Juliet Corbin. 1990. *Basics of Qualitative Research: Grounded Theory Procedures and Techniques.* Newbury Park, CA: Sage.

Tolich, Martin B. 1993. "Alienating and Liberating Emotions at Work: Supermarket Clerks' Performance of Customer Service." *Journal of Contemporary Ethnography* 22 (3): 361–81.

Tuominen, Mary C. 1998. "Motherhood and the Market: Mothering and Employment Opportunities among Mexican, African American, and Euro-American Family Day Care Workers." *Sociological Focus* 31 (1): 59–77.

———. 2003. *We Are Not Babysitters: Family Child Care Providers Redefine Work and Care.* New Brunswick, NJ: Rutgers University Press.

Twigg, Julia. 2000. "Carework as a Form of Body Work." *Aging and Society* 20 (4): 389–411.

Uttal, Lynet, and Mary Tuominen. 1999. "Tenuous Relationships: Exploitation, Emotion, and Racial Ethnic Significance in Paid Child Care Work." *Gender and Society* 13:758–80.

Voss, Kim, and Rachel Sherman. 2000. "Breaking the Iron Law of Oligarchy: Union Revitalization in the American Labor Movement." *American Journal of Sociology* 106 (2): 303–49.

Wakabayashi, Chizuko, and Katherine Donato. 2005. "The Consequences of Caregiving: Effects on Women's Employment and Earnings." *Population Research and Policy Review* 4:467–88.

———. 2006. "Does Caregiving Increase Poverty among Women in Later Life? Evidence from the Health and Retirement Survey." *Journal of Health and Social Behavior* 47 (3): 258–74.

Weaver, Adam. 2005. "Interactive Service Work and Performative Metaphors: The Case of the Cruise Industry." *Tourist Studies* 59 (1): 5–27.

Wellin, Chris. 2007. *Paid Caregiving for Older Adults with Serious or Chronic Illness: Ethnographic Perspectives, Evidence, and Implications for Training.* Washington DC: National Academies of Science.

Wharton, Amy. 1993. "The Affective Consequences of Service Work: Managing Emotions on the Job." *Work and Occupations* 20 (2): 205–32.

———. 1999. "The Psychosocial Consequences of Emotional Labor." *Annals of the American Academy* 561:158–76.

Wharton, Amy, and Rebecca J. Erickson. 1993. "Managing Emotions on the Job and at Home: Understanding the Consequences of Multiple Emotional Roles." *Academy of Management Review* 18 (3): 457–86.

Wharton, Carol S. 1996. "Making People Feel Good: Workers' Constructions of Meaning in Interactive Service Jobs." *Qualitative Sociology* 19 (2): 217–33.

Yamada, Yoshiko. 2002. "Profile of Home Care Aides, Nursing Home Aides, and Hospital Aides: Historical Changes and Data Recommendations." *Gerontologist* 42 (2): 199–206.

Zelizer, Viviana. 2005. *The Purchase of Intimacy.* Princeton, NJ: Princeton University Press.

Index

African Americans: and accusations of stealing, 126, 129; and the caring self, 22; demographics, 18, 31; and the sample, 17, 31, 126, 173. *See also* race and ethnicity

AFSCME (American Federation of the State, County, and Municipal Employees), 142, 179n4

age: aging, poverty and, 4; and differences in perception of fictive kinship bonds, 106; the sample and, 17, 173; and work ethic, 123–124

agencies: and aides performing medical procedures, 53; companionship exemption and, 164–165; discouragement of aide-client bonds, 63–64, 71–72, 97; and emotional labor, 61, 111, 160; feeling rules ignored by, 72, 159; "hands-off" approach of, 90–92; needs of, as prioritized, 61; non-profit, unionization of, 179n4; and training, lack of, 50–51, 54–55, 159. *See also* bureaucratic constraints; In-Home Supportive Services; private agencies

alienation of the self, 10–11, 33, 66, 76–78

Anderson, Leon, 107

Ashforth, Blake E., 10

Asians: and the caring self, 22, 130–132; and racism on the job, 126, 129; and the sample, 17, 126, 173

autonomy: ability to control emotionality on the job, 101–102; agency "hands-off" approach, 90–92; in context of interdependency, 101; and context of work, 92; by default, 95–96; functional, 92–96, 102; and home care, 21–22, 89, 92, 161; institutional care and lack of, 8, 92, 160–161; and job satisfaction, 34, 92, 95–96, 102; as key to caring self, 90, 92; relational, 96–102

Biklen, Molly, 166

boundary work, 117

bureaucratic constraints: as abstract, 56–57; assignment of hours inadequate, 61; and companionship needs, 57–58; de-skilling of the work, 55–56; liability issues and, 56; as relatively fewer in home-based care, 58–59; restrictions on scope of work, 56–58

compensation, inadequate: and length of workweek, 46; and number of clients per day, 46–47; and poverty of home care aides, 29–30, 116, 159
courtesy stigma, 125
custodial care, defined, 19

death of clients, 70–72, 101–102, 105, 159
demographics of clients, 18, 32, 126, 172. *See also* poverty of clients
demographics of home care aides: age, 17, 173; and crisis in long-term care, 4–5; education, 173; gender, 31, 173; national numbers, 7; racial/ethnic composition, 17, 18, 30–32, 126, 173; state comparisons of, 172; summary of, 17
Department of Labor, U.S., 165–166
de-skilling, 55–56
Diamond, Timothy, 8, 45, 130
dignity: and autonomy, 96, 102; boundary work and, 117; and the caring self, 135, 136; emotional capital and, 111; fictive kinship bonds producing, 22, 102; and identity work, 42; meaningful work and, 88–90, 175; social relations at work and, 88–89. *See also* caring self
Direct Care Alliance, 166, 177n2
direct care workers: burnout and turnover among, 33–34; as invisible, 157; invisible care gap of, 28. *See also* home care aides; institutional care
"dirty work" as stigma, 8, 161; and boundary work, 117–121; caring self and, 113, 135, 136, 161; and invisibility of direct care workers, 157
discrimination and racism on the job, 22, 31–32, 125–130, 132, 133–136; colorblind racism and, 132–133, 134, 135–136
division of labor: gendered, 6–7, 41–42, 109–110; racialized, 5, 30–32, 41, 134–135
Domestic Workers Bill of Rights, 180n1
Ducery, Ariel, 178n1

Ehrenreich, Barbara, 130
elder abuse, 122
emotional capital: caring trajectories and, 37, 38–39, 42, 43–44, 111; defined, 21, 35–36; emotional socialization and, 35–36; emotion as resource and, 34–35, 36; importance to job satisfaction, 158; lack of social/monetary value of, 21, 36, 111; as producing identity while also reinforcing inequality, 36, 158,

160; social location and, 35–36. *See also* caring self; caring trajectories
emotional connections to clients: and agencies "pulling" aides from clients, 59–60, 63; agency discouragement of, 63–64, 71–72, 97; as authentic, 10–11; boundaries sought as balance, 63–65; burnout and turnover and, 21; difficulty of disconnecting, 63; and job satisfaction, 14, 18, 34, 36, 42, 158; as motivation, 11; as skilled labor, 11, 42. *See also* caring self; companionship; fictive kinship bonds; uncompensated time/surplus care
emotional labor: and alienation of self, 10–11, 33, 66, 76–78; authentic emotion and, 10–11; autonomy and, 34; burnout and turnover and, 34, 65–68, 72, 158; companionship as labor, reconceptualization of, 166–169; context of, and job satisfaction, 10–11, 33, 34, 158; death of clients and, 70–72, 159; defined, 9–10, 33; domestic work distinguished from home care, 178n2; drug and alcohol use and, 68–69; emotion as resource and, 34–35; and lack of clear boundaries between work and home, 67–68, 106; mental health issues and, 69–70; overextension and, 30, 63, 65, 90, 160; overinvestment and, 11, 66, 159–160; and research, lack of, 33; as source of both inequality and identity, 36, 158, 160; talking about, importance of, 22; as unrecognized by agencies and policymakers, 61, 111. *See also* burnout and turnover; dignity; emotional capital; feeling rules
emotional overinvestment, 11, 66, 159–160
emotional proletariat, 9, 10, 32–36, 159
ethic of care, personal, 8, 99, 115, 160–161. *See also* speed-up of work
Executive Order 23S, 145–147, 179nn3-4

Fair Home Health Care Act, 165
Fair Labor Standards Act (FLSA), 23, 164–166, 168, 177n2, 180n2
families of clients: burnout and dealing with, 160; and emotional labor, 72–76; fictive kinship bonds encouraged by, 104–105; as paid caregivers, 142, 145, 174, 180n5; unable or unwilling to provide unpaid care, 7, 73–74; as uncaring, boundary making of aides toward, 117–121

CPSIA information can be obtained
at www.ICGtesting.com
Printed in the USA
LVHW042134061218
599510LV00001B/131